Acute Illness Management

SAGE has been part of the global academic community since 1965, supporting high quality research and learning that transforms society and our understanding of individuals, groups and cultures. SAGE is the independent, innovative, natural home for authors, editors and societies who share our commitment and passion for the social sciences.

Find out more at: **www.sagepublications.com**

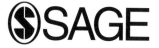

Acute Illness Management

Chris Mulryan

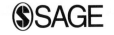

Los Angeles | London | New Delhi
Singapore | Washington DC

SAGE Publications Ltd
1 Oliver's Yard
55 City Road
London EC1Y 1SP

SAGE Publications Inc.
2455 Teller Road
Thousand Oaks, California 91320

SAGE Publications India Pvt Ltd
B 1/I 1 Mohan Cooperative Industrial Area
Mathura Road
New Delhi 110 044

SAGE Publications Asia-Pacific Pte Ltd
33 Pekin Street #02-01
Far East Square
Singapore 048763

Library of Congress Control Number: 2010935083

British Library Cataloguing in Publication data

A catalogue record for this book is available from the British Library

ISBN 978-1-84787-955-4
ISBN 978-1-84787-956-1 (pbk)

Knowledge and best practice in this area are subject to constant change. Readers are advised to keep themselves up to date on the most current information available in relation to the procedures outlined in this book. It is the responsibility of the practitioner using their own clinical judgment, information and experience of the patient to determine the best treatment for each individual patient including all appropriate safety precautions. Neither SAGE nor the Author assumes nor shall have any liability for injury and/or damage to persons or property and/or death directly or indirectly arising out of or related to any of the material in this book or otherwise.

Typeset by C&M Digitals (P) Ltd, Chennai, India
Printed by MPG Books Group, Bodmin, Cornwall
Printed on paper from sustainable resources

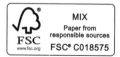

Contents

Dedication and thanks

To
Marc Alexander Mulryan RIP 1979–1996
(Mr Tartleaf, as it is a special occasion)
and
those who have suffered harm needlessly for the want of better acute care

Special thanks
Many people have helped to bring this text to fruition. Special thanks are due to Zoe Elliot-Fawcet for commissioning the book. Dr Clive Taylor for his amazing support, encouragement and his critical eye. He read countless drafts and without him this book would not have made the press. Dr Lavinia Norton for teaching me so well. Lara Mulryan for the images that she has contributed. Alison Poyner, Emma Paterson and Emma Milman for their patience and support throughout this project. Katie Forsythe for guiding me effortlessly through the production process. Others at SAGE who have worked to bring this text to the shelf.

About the author

Chris Mulryan is senior lecturer at the University of Bolton where he teaches on a variety of programmes including the MSc in Advanced Practice, BSc in Health and Social Care and the Diploma in Paramedic Practice. In addition to this he also contributes the popular multidisciplinary continuing professional development framework provided by the university. Chris's academic interests are mainly concerned with patient safety and how expert clinical care contributes to this. To this end he is keen to teach about the body in a rigorous yet accessible way so that health professional have a developed understanding of how diseases affect the body and how medical therapies work to better or restore health.

List of abbreviations

°C	Degree Celsius
ABCDE	Airway, Breathing, Circulation, Disability, Exposure
ABG	Arterial Blood Gas
ACE	Angiotensin Converting Enzyme
ACS	Acute Coronary Syndrome
AED	Automated External Defibrillator
AF	Atrial Fibrillation
ALTE	Acute Life Threatening Event
ARDS	Acute (Adult) Respiratory Distress Syndrome
ATP	Adenosine Triphosphate
AV	Atrioventricular
AVPU	Alert, Voice, Pain, Unresponsive
BiPAP	Bi-level Positive Airway Pressure
BMA	British Medical Association
BP	Blood Pressure
bpm	Beats per Minute
CAD	Coronary Artery Disease
CCOT	Critical Care Outreach Team
CPAP	Continuous Positive Airway Pressure
CPR	Cardiopulmonary Resuscitation
DIC	Disseminated Intravascular Coagulopathy
DNAR	Do Not Attempt Resuscitation
ECG	Electrocardiograph
EWS	Early Warning Score
FiO2%	Fraction Inspired Oxygen
GTN	Glyceryl Trinitrate
HONK	Hyperosmolar Non-Ketotic State
ID	Internal Diameter
IO	Intraosseous
IPPV	Intermittent Positive Pressure Ventilation
ITU	Intensive Therapy Unit
IV	Intra Venous

K	Potassium
kPa	Kilopascal
LEP	Legal, Ethical, Professional
LMA	Laryngeal Mask Airway
LPM	Litres per Minute
LT	Laryngeal Tube
MAP	Mean Arterial Pressure
MET	Medical Emergency Team
MI	Myocardial infarction
mℓ	Millilitres
mmHg	Millimetres of mercury
mmol/L	Millimole per litre
Na	Sodium
NPA	Nasopharyngeal Airway
NSR	Normal Sinus Rhythm
NSTEMI	Non-S-T Elevation Myocardial Infarction
OPA	Oropharyngeal Airway
PAC	Premature Atrial Contraction
PaCO$_2$	Partial Pressure of Carbon Dioxide in Arterial Blood
PaO$_2$	Partial Pressure of Oxygen in Arterial Blood
PEA	Pulseless Electrical Activity
PEFR	Peak Expiratory Flow Rate
pH	(*potenz* Hydrogen) Measure of Acidity
PJC	Premature Junctional Contraction
PSA	Patient Stability Assessment
PVC	Premature Ventricular Contraction
RCB	Red Blood Cell
ROSC	Return of Spontaneous Circulation
SA	Sinoatrial
SaO$_2$	Saturation of Oxygen in Arterial Blood
SIRS	Systemic Inflammatory Response Syndrome
STEMI	S-T Elevation Myocardial Infarction
SVT	Supraventricular Tachycardia
UAP	Unstable Angina Pectoris
VF	Ventricular Fibrillation
VT	Ventricular Tachycardia
WBC	White Blood Cell

Introduction

'To live through an impossible situation, you don't need the reflexes of a grand prix driver, the muscles of a Hercules or the mind of an Einstein. You simply need to know what to do.' (Greenbank, 2003)

Nowhere is this statement truer than in the care of those who become acutely ill. Unfortunately, however, health professionals often report feeling poorly prepared for the role that they may be called on to play should a patient become acutely ill. In response to these common concerns, this book attempts to demystify the topic of acute illness management in order to provide health professionals with a more developed understanding of the key topics that underpin the safe care of those who are at risk of becoming or who actually become acutely ill.

Specifically this book aims to provide an accessible yet authoritative account of the main reasons why and how patients become acutely ill and how to recognise deterioration in a patient's condition early in the course of the disease process, and finally an explanation of the key strategies used in the management of patients who are acutely ill. Underpinning this are chapters that address the legal, ethical and professional issues and the more psycho-social aspects of care.

The intention of this book is not to drill you in following protocols, but to develop your understanding of what occurs physiologically during an episode of acute illness so that this basic knowledge can inform a problem-solving approach to care. This in turn will assist you in understanding acute illness so that you can both avert deterioration and respond to it when it occurs.

The direction this book takes is to first explain what acute illness is and the various ways through which it can develop. This then leads on to a description of the physiological mechanisms that maintain homeostasis and how these are challenged at times of acute illness, which helps in understanding the changes that occur in the body during an episode of acute illness. Next, this foundation is related to the care that is provided to individual patients at the varying stages of acute illness by considering the rationale for the different assessment and treatment options that are utilised in the care of the acutely ill person. The book aims to make you think in an investigative way when assessing patients so that you can not only recognise abnormal clinical signs, but also explain those findings and what their implications are for the patient and their care. Finally, you are encouraged to instigate appropriate management of the acutely ill patient, again while being able to justify why this care is needed and what it hopes to achieve. Whereas this approach will bring benefits for patients, it is also hoped that this text will help to make the care of the acutely ill less of something that brings about anxiety and more of something that you are confident about and find rewarding to provide.

In short this book aims to provide an introductory guide to the key components of caring for those who are at risk of becoming acutely ill. It intends to be a kind of survival guide for health professionals who may become involved in the care of acutely ill patients, which in reality is any patient in any clinical setting.

How to use this book

This book has been designed to introduce the reader to the principles of caring for the acutely ill. As such it is intended that the book is read in its entirety as each section deals with a different aspect of the assessment and management of the acutely ill patient. This book takes a generic approach to the subject of caring for the acutely ill without trying to link findings to a specific diagnosis. It focuses on recognising and correcting abnormalities of physiology that are common to all medical and surgical specialities involving adults. This approach enables you to deduce what is occurring within a patient physiologically and then be able to react to this without investing time in working out a specific diagnosis.

To help you learn about acute illness this book has been organised in a way that helps to integrate theory into your practice. Each chapter commences with a set of chapter aims. These are points that you should know after reading the chapter and completing the exercises within it. When you start reading each chapter be clear about what it is you are expected to achieve from reading the chapter and then at the end of the chapter go back to the chapter aims and consider whether you think that you have achieved them.

Throughout this book you will find various activities that you are encouraged to undertake if you are to generate the most learning from this book. Some of these exercises will be reflective and others will require you to do things in your practice setting. Both are equally important to developing your acute care skills. Each chapter also concludes with some self-assessment questions. These are designed to help you judge whether you have developed a good grasp of the topic or if there are gaps in your knowledge that you should try to address.

After reading this book you may wish to enhance your knowledge in a way that is more specific in terms of the conditions that people in your area of practice present with. This is a sensible step and one that is to be encouraged. That said, it is important to recognise that in the initial stages of managing those who become acutely ill the process of management is largely generic and the systematic approach that is proposed in this book should still be followed.

It is sincerely hoped that you find this book both enjoyable and informative. Probably more importantly it is hoped that you find this book useful in improving the care that you provide to patients who suffer the misfortune of becoming acutely ill.

Chris Mulryan

1

Acute illness management: an overview

Chapter aims

By the end of this chapter you should be able to:

- Define what acute illness is
- Explain how acute illness typically develops in patients
- Identify some deficiencies in how acutely ill patients are recognised and managed
- Describe some potential ways through which acute care can be enhanced
- Review your own practice with regard to acute illness management and identify any learning needs that you may have

Acutely ill individuals can present in all healthcare settings and thus every health professional needs to have the knowledge and skills necessary to respond to this group of patients. In practice, this means that all health professionals must be able to recognise those who are at risk of becoming acutely ill and take early action to stabilise them in order to avert further deterioration.

Defining acute illness

Before going any further with the discussion of acute illness, it is important establish what exactly acute illness is. On reviewing the literature, it is difficult to find one definition of acute illness that would suitably cover all patients in all specialities. What is easy to locate is a definition of the term 'acute', which is synonymous with illness that is rapid in onset, severe and short lived. The term 'acute illness' therefore describes patients who have rapidly become ill with a severe condition that may be life-threatening, with a degree of reversibility to it.

The inclusion of the term 'rapid' can be a little confusing as it conjures images of sudden collapse and as such requires further clarification. There is evidence that patients who suffer cardiac arrest have significant changes in their clinical observations for up to 24 hours before the cardiac arrest occurs (Hodgetts et al., 2002). This suggests that for many patients there is a period of acute illness that precedes the cardiac arrest. In this context, the term rapid therefore encompasses a gradual and insidious decline that occurs progressively over hours as opposed to weeks. While cardiac arrest, defined by the cessation of breathing and absence of cardiac output, represents an end point in this decline, there is a significant window of opportunity to intervene prior to arriving at this critical end point, which potentially allows cardiac arrest to be averted in some patients and morbidity reduced in others.

It should then be possible to define this time period of acute illness that precedes many cardiac arrests. To describe this phase of illness, where the patient is maximally physiologically disarranged, I shall use the term acute life-threatening event (ALTE). While ALTE is more difficult to define than cardiac arrest, it represents a period of time prior to cardiac arrest when a patient requires emergency resuscitation to avert cardiac arrest or other serious complications of an ALTE. The aim of acute illness management is then to detect those who are en route to, or have arrived at, an ALTE and to treat them rapidly and effectively before complications can occur.

Acute illness: a physiological disarrangement

Illness is something that spans a continuum of different clinical states that a patient may find themselves in; Figure 1.1 illustrates the regions of this spectrum. For most patients who become ill, the self-limiting nature of the illness and ability to self-repair confines the illness to the minor illness bracket. For others where the cause of the illness is more serious or the person's ability to self-repair is limited, they will progress on to the serious illness bracket. When this occurs the body will attempt to compensate for the illness state that has been encountered in an effort to maintain homeostasis. However, the body's ability to compensate for illness is limited, and illnesses,

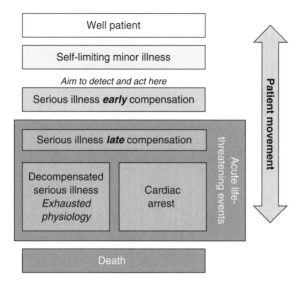

FIGURE 1.1   *The spectrum of acute illness.*

if severe, can exhaust the compensatory mechanisms of the body and bring about a massive physiological disarrangement. At the same time the activation of the compensatory mechanism places additional demands on an already diseased body and this in itself can further worsen the physiological disarrangement experienced by the patient. In some cases of acute illness it is in fact the body's own healing mechanism that bring about the illness state.

As the patient moves along the spectrum, from a point of wellness to a point where they are at risk of death, they will experience mounting physiological disarrangement. The further a patient moves along the spectrum of acute illness, the more difficult it is to correct their ailing physiology and the more likely it is that they will endure heightened morbidity and mortality. The speed at which a patient will progress along this spectrum is dependent on the actual cause of the disease; for some the progression will be quite slow but for others the progression may occur in quick succession with a small minority experiencing a sudden shift from a well patient state to cardiac arrest.

Acute illness is in simple terms a problem with a person's physiology that interrupts or hinders the factors that would normally regulate homeostasis (Chapter 2). There are many factors that can interfere with homeostasis, and while it is beyond the scope of this text to explore each and every one of the disease processes that can result in acute illness, Chapter 2 will endeavour to explain some most important physiological concepts that underpin the development and management of acute illness. Example causes of acute illness are provided in Box 1.1.

BOX 1.1 Examples of acute illnesses

Airway obstruction, resulting in difficulty in breathing and ultimately hypoxia

- Loss of muscle tone/gag reflex
- Vomit
- Foreign body
- Swelling of the airway

Breathing problems, resulting in hypoxia and possibly acidic blood

- Acute asthma
- Exacerbation of chronic obstructive pulmonary disease
- Pneumonia
- Carbon monoxide poisoning
- Pneumothorax/plural effusion

Circulatory problems, resulting in shock and possibly acidic blood

- Myocardial infarction
- Heart failure
- Vomiting and diarrhoea causing dehydration, blood loss, other fluid loss
- A problem with the heart's rhythm (arrhythmia)

Kidney problems (renal failure)

- Too much fluid in the body (hypervolaemia/fluid overload)
- Too little fluid in the body (hypovolaemia)
- Altered electrolyte balance, particularly of sodium, potassium and calcium
- Problems with the regulation of acid in the blood
- Problems with blood pressure (hypertension/hypotension)
- Problems with red blood cell production (anaemia)

Problems with how acute illness is managed

It is now well recognised that acutely ill patients are not always well managed. Indeed a study by McQuillan et al. (1998) demonstrated that poor quality acute care not only occurred, but also that where patients were subjected to poor quality care either by not being recognised as acutely ill soon enough or not being managed correctly that there was a dramatic worsening in a patient's chances of surviving the episode. McQuillan et al. (1998) discovered that patients were approximately 20% more likely to die when they were the recipients of poor quality care prior to intensive care unit (ITU) admission. Hodgetts et al. (2002) also demonstrated that an estimated 23,000 otherwise preventable in-hospital cardiac arrests occur in the UK each year as a result of poor quality acute care. These both shocking and saddening statistics are made worse when one considers that most of the variables that lead to poor patient outcomes relate to basic facets of care such as appropriately interpreting nursing observations, maintaining an adequate fluid balance, providing tailored oxygen therapy and maintaining a patient's airway and breathing (National Confidential Enquiry into Patient Outcome and Death, 2005).

While the picture that has thus far been painted of the state of acute illness management is quite a dismal one, a positive point to bear in mind is that many of the failings are readily reversible. This sets forth a challenge for health professionals to identify areas of poor practice and put in place plans to correct it.

Improving the response to the acutely ill

Several strategies have been proposed to improve the response to the acutely ill. These have included the use of early warning scores (EWS), early goal-directed therapies and improved education for those charged with responsibility for detecting acute illness and managing it. Following the development of EWS systems (Morgan et al., 1997; Stubbe et al., 2001) the National Institute for Health and Clinical Excellence issued guidelines on how to monitor people who are acutely ill and how to act once deterioration has been detected (NICE, 2007). These guidelines advocate the use of EWS systems for patients cared for in hospital.

EWS systems are essentially decision support tools which allow the identification of those who are at risk of deterioration. Most do this by setting reference ranges for physiological observations that are usually taken in the clinical environment. When these observations deviate from the reference range, a score is applied. When the score reaches a certain threshold, a specific action is required as dictated by local protocols. The 2007 NICE guidance on the acutely ill in hospital recommends that the scores generated by EWS are classified as either low, medium or high and the clinical response that a patient receives is directed by this classification. These classifications are set locally and will vary according to the EWS tool used, of which there are many, with different thresholds for action set by local advisors. This potentially introduces an inequality, as patients seen in different hospitals may be classified differently even when they present with clinically identical observations. To combat this situation, the Royal

College of Physicians proposed the development of an NHS early warning score, to be known as the NEW score (RCP, 2007). Indeed Prytherch et al. (2010) have recently developed and validated a scoring system that holds significant promise to standardise EWS.

While EWS systems play an important role and act as an enhancement to previous practice, their use is only a small part of the answer to the problems surrounding the care of the acutely ill. As with all protocols, they are designed to be used by thinking people. To illustrate the importance of thought, consider the observations listed and try to answer the questions in Box 1.2.

BOX 1.2   Observations to consider

- Respiratory rate: 18 breaths per min
- Pulse: 82 beats per min in normal sinus rhythm
- Blood pressure: 112/84 mmHg
- SaO$_2$: 96%

Questions

1 Look at the observations and map them against an EWS that you use locally.
2 Would you be concerned about a patient with these observations?
3 What, if anything, would lead you to have concerns about a patient with these observations?

On most of the currently available EWS systems the values in Box 1.2 would score zero, indicating that the patient was well and no trigger would be raised to command a clinical response to this patient. Now, if your patient is James Anderson, a 19-year-old man presenting to you after sustaining an ankle injury during a game of football, no loss of consciousness (LOC), no past medical history (PMH), who takes no medications – prescribed, over the counter or illicit – and has no allergies, then there is probably little to worry about physiologically based on the limited observations given. If, however, it was his grandfather Andrew Anderson, a 78-year-old, who was taking beta-blockers and angiotensin-converting enzyme (ACE) inhibitors and had had a myocardial infarction in 1997, a positive history for transient ischaemic attacks with type 2 diabetes, micro-albuminurea and was normally hypertensive with a blood pressure of 188/96 mmHg who presented to you with ripping chest pain, then the clinical circumstances would be quite different. Although Andrew has a EWS of zero he is likely to be profoundly haemodynamically unstable. The effects of beta-blockade and ACE inhibition have reduced his ability to compensate and hence he shows no signs of compensation in the observations given. The drop in his blood pressure is significant and worrisome, and taken with his history and presenting symptoms warrants immediate resuscitation and further investigation, ideally in a critical care area. From this simple case illustration, it can be seen that more than a tick-box system is needed if the acutely ill are to be reliably identified and managed.

Coupled with the ability to recognise the acutely ill patient is the need to manage them once detected. One strategy that can assist with doing this in an organised and responsive manner is early goal-directed resuscitation. Resuscitation is something that many solely associate with the response to a person who has had either a cardiac or respiratory arrest. Cardiopulmonary resuscitation or CPR is only one type of resuscitation, and resuscitation is a term with much wider utility. Simply put, resuscitation refers to restoring something to a normal state. Resuscitation can therefore be used to describe many other interventions that are designed to restore a person to a normal state. As such, resuscitative efforts can take place long before a person has a cardiac arrest and in many circumstances before the person has become acutely ill and experiences an ALTE. Terms such as fluid resuscitation and homeostatic resuscitation are examples of this, where the goal of resuscitation is not to restart a person's arrested heart, but to restore either a normal fluid balance or some other collection of physiological parameters that have become disarranged by the development of an illness state. The ultimate aim of this type of resuscitation is to prevent the development of an ALTE, averting the possibility of cardiac arrest and ultimately attempting to restore health.

Traditionally, care of the acutely ill individual was escalated at the point of gross abnormality in a person's physiology or where cardiac arrest had occurred; this is a critical oversight as any resuscitative efforts are much less likely to succeed at this late stage. Having established that cardiac arrest is often a preventable condition, it is important that resuscitation is started early and long before any gross abnormality occurs in a person's physiology if the best possible outcome is to be achieved.

The term 'goal-directed' resuscitation involves tailoring treatments given to achieve specific outcomes. For example consider how oxygen and intravenous fluid is administered to the acutely ill patient. It would theoretically be possible to provide the same treatment to all patients, as indeed most patients who become acutely ill will require both oxygen and intravenous fluid; however, this approach would result in some patients being overtreated while others were undertreated. The concept of goal-directed resuscitation sees that treatment is given in a sufficient quantity to achieve a specific aim; for oxygen therapy this could be maintenance of the saturation of arterial oxygen between 94% and 98% or for intravenous fluid to keep the systolic blood pressure at 90 mmHg. Treatment in a goal-directed approach is given in an escalating pattern until the desired goal is achieved. Using this approach ensures that each patient receives the minimum yet most appropriate level of treatment needed to provide optimal support to their failing physiology. Goal-directed therapy has been a feature of intensive care medicine for many years now and its expansion to the non-ITU setting is timely and wholly appropriate for the initial management and stabilisation of the acutely ill patient (Rivers, 2001). When employing goal-directed therapy it is important though not to underestimate the severity of a patient's illness. The use of medical therapies to artificially support homeostasis in a person with failing physiology can restore blood pressure, oxygen saturations, etc., to a normal or near normal range. Where this is the case it is important to recognise that while homeostasis is being maintained, it is being achieved artificially and the person while more stable is dependent on the medical interventions that are stabilising them; however, the patient remains seriously unwell despite normal or near normal vital signs. This point not only illustrates the ability of goal-directed therapies to temporarily repair abnormal physiology but also shows the importance of factoring in the impact of any therapies that a patient might be in receipt of when making decisions about their stability.

Reflecting on your own acute illness management practice

While providing good quality care for a person who has become acutely ill is one of the most rewarding jobs that any health professional can undertake, it is also an activity that can provoke much anxiety for the caregiver. Some health professionals have even gone so far as to report overt fear at the mere thought of having to perform CPR (O'Donnell, 1990). While the exact reasons for this are likely to be multifactorial, a perceived lack of adequate preparation for the roles that health professionals are called upon to play has been cited as a problem (O'Donnell, 1990; Hamilton, 2005). This is an important observation, as improving the education of health professionals in the discipline of acute illness management could ultimately be a fundamental part of the solution to the problems with acute care that have been cited previously. This is particularly true when one considers that even if the acutely ill are identified using a scoring system, staff must be prepared and equipped to respond to the physiological changes that have been detected. An education that enhances the ability of health professionals to both recognise and respond to the acutely ill patient is then a recurring theme and an important backdrop to the care that people receive.

A report by the Resuscitation Council (UK) and Intercollegiate Board for Training in Intensive Care Medicine (2005), the 'ACUTE initiative', identifies a range of competencies that are essential for providing good quality acute care. The ACUTE initiative report suggests that these competencies be present in all doctors as they leave medical school. While this report is primarily aimed at undergraduate doctors, the principles of the report can be easily extrapolated to other health professions; for example if a doctor is expected to perform a procedure then others should be able to assist with it. Likewise, some areas of care can be shared between different professions. The domains identified in the ACUTE initiative are listed in Box 1.3.

BOX 1.3 Domains of competence suggested by the ACUTE initiative

- Airway and oxygenation
- Breathing and ventilation
- Circulation
- Confusion and coma
- Drugs, therapeutics and protocols
- Clinical examination, monitoring and investigations
- Teamworking, organisation and communication
- Patient and societal needs
- Trauma
- Equipment
- Infection and inflammation

Any education programme that is designed to prepare health professionals for managing the acutely ill and taking part in a resuscitation attempt needs to function on a number of levels and will ideally consist of several distinct phases rather than being an isolated short course. The aim of the programme should be to shift thinking and to bring about competence. To do this successfully, educational programmes will need to ensure that a robust body of knowledge is developed. Alongside this, participants will need to become competent in performing a number of practical skills. Finally, participants must be taught how to use the knowledge and skills that they have gained in simulated clinical environments. Ideally, this should be augmented by attendance at ALTEs and cardiac arrests as an

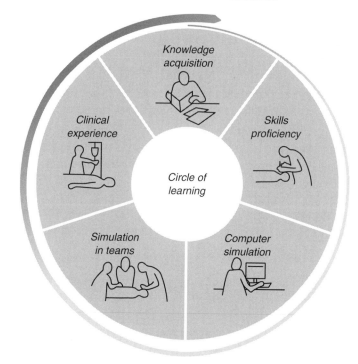

FIGURE 1.2   *The circle of learning.*
Reproduced with the kind permission of Laerdal Medical.

observer with the resuscitation team. This method of developing acute care skills is summarised by Laerdal (2010) in their circle of learning (Figure 1.2). Unfortunately many educational programmes still fall short of incorporating all of the aspects advocated by Laerdal, and as a result provide arguably inadequate preparation based on current knowledge.

The stages of learning

Knowledge is what you know about a given subject. Largely, in acute care there are known right and wrong answers to questions that relate to anatomy, physiology and pathology. A measure of your knowledge is therefore the extent to which you can reproduce these known answers and explain where this knowledge came from. Having this knowledge will enable you to work out why you are seeing what you are seeing and why you need to react to it in a given manner. 'There is no shortcut to knowledge' and never has a truer word been uttered. Learning all you need to know about acute illness will be time-consuming without a doubt, but it is also likely to be life-saving when considered in the light of the above data.

Skills can be described as the practical things that you do as a part of your practice. This could be something like assembling a bag-valve mask device or performing chest compressions. As with knowledge, there is often a right and wrong way to deploy skills. Getting a clinical skill wrong can be profoundly dangerous to the patient to the extent of costing them their life. Here, the aphorism 'practice makes perfect' is apt. You should never be expected to become competent in a skill such as CPR after having a one-minute trial on a manikin in an unrealistic environment with a large group of co-learners. It is totally inconceivable to imagine that this will adequately prepare you for practice. To learn clinical skills effectively, the following ten steps to learning are proposed:

1   You are taught (or gain in another way) the complete set of knowledges needed to practise the skill safely.
2   You demonstrate that you have the knowledge to safely use the skill.
3   You observe a demonstration of the skill in a safe (simulated) environment.
4   You practise the skill in a safe and supervised environment time and again until you feel confident.
5   You are formally assessed by a competent person in a safe patient-free environment as being able to perform the skill.
6   You watch the skill being performed on a real patient.
7   You perform the skill on real patients under direct supervision several times.
8   You are formally assessed performing the skill on real patients and demonstrate competence.
9   You are allowed to practise the skill independently.
10 You keep your knowledge and skills up to date and accept responsibility for performing the skill safely.

For some skills, say the performance of CPR, it may be difficult to fulfil the above taxonomy in its entirety due to a lack of patients with cardiac arrest, and as such a more robust simulated assessment can be organised.

Having developed both the knowledge and skills, the next step is to be able to combine them in a therapeutic sequence that will benefit patients. For the sake of argument, this will be called integration. Most acute care requires a number of simple, distinct skills to be brought together by a thinking individual and it is this component of care that is the most difficult in which to educate people. At this stage you must be able to recognise when you need to react and use your knowledge and skills. You also need to recognise when it is inappropriate to react. It is most probably the ability to integrate and react appropriately that is most critical in responding to the acutely ill.

Thanks to developments in the way training manikins are designed, it is now possible to create simulated environments with simulated patients, which can be compared with flight simulators that are used to train pilots. The benefit of these simulated environments is largely that professionals can practise their skills in a realistic environment without risk of harming a patient and develop excellent skills in integration.

Assessment is an essential component of any educational programme. The assessments should test each aspect of preparation. Assessment is needed at the end of each stage of the previously described ten steps to developing clinical skills. The assessments should test knowledge, practical skills and finally how you make use of this knowledge and these skills as a part of integration while reacting to simulated scenarios. Along with this formal assessment it is also helpful to self-audit your own practice. The results of this audit can then inform further learning that you may wish to undertake. To aid you in this audit process try undertaking the activities in Boxes 1.4 and 1.5.

BOX 1.4   Confidence in caring for the acutely ill

Many people are apprehensive about caring for people who are acutely ill or have had a cardiac arrest. In order to improve your confidence and performance it is important to audit your skills. Read through the list below and rank each of the topics with how you feel about it. Use the following descriptors: very confident; confident; not confident; my practice could be unsafes.

1   The normal values of basic physiological observations for all patient groups
2   The ability to interpret a person's observations in the light of their current circumstances
3   Predict who is at risk of deterioration
4   Open a person's airway
5   Insert a laryngeal mask
6   Assist with intubation
7   Assess the work of breathing
8   Assess for the presence of respiratory failure
9   Examine a person's chest
10   Assess the effectiveness of circulation
11   Explain fluid distribution within the body
12   Assess a person's blood volume status
13   Perform external chest compressions
14   Perform defibrillation
15   Check emergency equipment

When you have read this book, repeat this exercise and see if your views have changed and try to identify any areas you still need to learn more about. If there are areas you need to learn more about, try make a time-bound plan to assist you in organising this learning.

BOX 1.5 Practice in your work setting

Think about your workplace and make two lists. The first list should be all the things that you think are good about how your workplace responds to the needs of the acutely ill. The second list should be made up of things that you think are not good and could be improved.

Keep these lists and come back to them when you have read this book in its entirety. Then consider if you still think the lists are correct and if there is anything that you want to change in them. If you have discovered anything that you think is not good or could be improved, think about how you could go about making changes in your workplace to improve patient care and discuss these with your manager. You could then write a reflection on this and keep it in your professional portfolio as evidence of practice development activity.

Conclusion

Caring for acutely ill patients is often challenging, sometimes stressful, yet rewarding for health professionals. Unfortunately, some of the current practice that surrounds the care received by this group of patients is not always optimal; in turn this leads to an avoidable increase in morbidity and mortality for those who become acutely ill and do not receive appropriate care. Problems that have been identified with the current approach to the acutely ill patient have been associated with patients deteriorating unnoticed and, when deterioration was noticed, failing to provide an appropriate response. That said, most of the failures in care often relate to simple aspects of observation and basic management of a patient's physiology. As the aspects of care that need to be improved are simple, it is relatively easy to employ some basic learning and use a systematic approach to the acutely ill patient in order to improve practice and optimise the patient's experience and outcome. Strategies such as the implementation of early warning systems and goal-directed therapy can help, but these must be supported by thinking professionals who can adjust their judgement to take into account the individual patient's circumstances.

Much of effective acute illness management is centred around understanding the physiology of the human body, how this is altered at times of illness and how this can be supported with medical therapies in a structured and organised way. Readers are encouraged to keep this fact in view as they progress through this text. The reminder of this book hopes to assist practitioners to build on this knowledge of physiology and how this relates to the development of acute illness in a given organ system and the body as a whole. Linked to this is a physiological understanding of how illness develops and how the strategies that are commonly employed in the early stages of recognising and managing the acutely ill patient operate. Readers are also encouraged to be open to suggestions of new ways of thinking about activities that are delivered in practice and to be self-critical of their own practice, in order to learn from this and in turn take action to improve the care received by acutely ill patients.

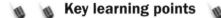

Key learning points

- All health professionals, no matter what their area of practice, should be capable of recognising the acutely ill patient and initiating resuscitation.
- Acute illness occurs when a person's ability to maintain homeostasis is challenged.
- Acute illness is a spectrum of stages ranging from minor illness to pre-terminal conditions.
- Many acutely ill patients deteriorate unnoticed and receive suboptimal care.
- Suboptimal care often relates to simple aspects of patient management.
- Suboptimal care results in significantly higher morbidity and mortality.
- Many cardiac arrests that occur are preventable.
- Early goal-directed resuscitation can improve outcomes.
- Education and training can improve both confidence and outcomes.
- Professionals should continually audit their own skills and undertake updating activity as necessary.

Further reading

National Confidential Enquiry into Patient Outcome and Death (2005) *An Acute Problem. A Report of the National Confidential Enquiry into Patient Outcome and Death* (2005). London: NCEPOD.
This document reports on the problems that surround acute care in hospitals with some important results that highlight a number of inadequacies.

National Institute for Health and Clinical Excellence (2007) *Acutely Ill Patients in Hospital: Recognition of and Response to Acute Illness in Adults in Hospital.* London: NICE.
This document outlines the approach to the assessment of the acutely ill in hospitalised patients in the light of the National Confidential Enquiry into Patient Outcome and Death, which revealed a poor standard of care for the acutely ill.

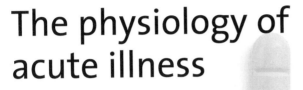

2

The physiology of acute illness

Chapter aims

By the end of this chapter you should be able to:

- Define homeostasis and outline the actions that the body takes to maintain homeostasis
- Describe in basic terms the systems of the body that control cell energy production, fluid distribution, inflammation and acid–base balance
- Identify insults that can affect the body and describe how the body reacts
- Explain the concepts of compensated and decompensated illness
- Relate the changes in physiology that occur during acute illness to the basic observations that health professionals make
- Recognise a need to work in a goal-directed way to support the physiology of those who are acutely ill

During periods of acute illness, a person's physiology changes in order that they can respond to the injury or insult that their body faces. Clinically, it is these changes in physiology – the compensatory mechanisms – that we as health professionals look for when assessing people and making conclusions about a patient's stability. All treatments that are used in the resuscitation of an acutely ill individual aim to correct the disarrangement of basic physiology and support the body in an effort to restore homeostasis.

Given that physiology, patient assessment and management are directly linked in a close relationship, it is fundamentally necessary for those caring for people who are at risk of becoming acutely ill to understand the physiological changes that occur during an episode of acute illness. Such an understanding enables health professionals to look for evidence of these changes in patients and take appropriate goal-directed action to address them. This chapter will explain these basic, yet fundamental concepts of physiology and pathophysiology in order that you, a health professional charged with caring for those who are at risk of becoming acutely ill, can do so in an informed manner. While many readers will want to progress rapidly to subsequent chapters that deal with the more practical aspects of managing the acutely ill, this chapter provides an invaluable foundation, and time given over to learning the content of this chapter will reap many rewards, not only while reading further chapters in this book but also in practice.

The basics

Before you can understand the assessment and management of the ill adult, it is necessary to understand some basic biological concepts that underpin how the body functions and reacts to stressors in a way that leads to the development of an illness state. Many of these basic concepts are common to all disease processes that occur within the body and as such make for essential learning. While it is not within the scope of this text to provide a full introduction to pathology, the components of disease development that are important features of acute illness will be outlined in order that you can use this to inform your practice.

The human body is an amazingly complex entity. On a purely biological level, one can view the body as distinct parts, each with a specific function. While to some degree this view of the body is correct and assists in our understanding of the body, it is of paramount importance to recognise that each individual component interacts throughout in a kind of cause and effect relationship and thus a simple change in one part of the body can result in a chain of events which have the potential to result in both positive and negative outcomes for the patient.

Individual cells are the functional building blocks of the body and as living organisms we invest great effort in ensuring that our cells remain healthy. Essentially, this means that each of our cells must be constantly supplied with the components needed to nourish the cell, and waste products must be removed. When cells are not supplied with the needed components or waste is not removed, injury to the cell can occur and, if severe, cell death can ensue. Inappropriate cell death is in truth death to a part of the body and if cell death is widespread then serious consequences for the person as a whole will follow. In response to cell death, the body has a system that serves to limit the impact that this has on the body physiologically. This is called the inflammatory process. However, when injury to cells is widespread, these protective mechanisms can overwhelm and turn against the body that they are intended to protect. This chapter will start out by examining how cells are kept healthy. It will then move on look at ways to prevent and detect cell injury. Finally the chapter will discuss some of the common changes that can occur in a body that contains cells which have become injured or died.

Homeostasis

Human beings are known as homeotherms. In essence this means that we are warm-blooded creatures, each having a protected internal environment that is largely independent of or resistant to changes in the outside environment. Put more simply, humans can maintain their body temperature in cold weather and keep moisture inside the body when its surroundings are extremely dry. Having a protected internal environment has a number of advantages and disadvantages for humans. When the body cannot maintain this internal environment, cells are harmed and illness develops.

The most significant point that needs to be understood when contemplating the body's internal environment is how very tightly controlled it is and how a slight deficiency or excess of chemicals within the body can result in a dramatic physiological disarrangement, the result of which can be severe systemic illness and potentially death. In order to avert physiological disarrangement, the healthy individual has a number of automatic mechanisms which ensure that there remains tight physiological control and that chemical concentrations within the body stay within their defined reference (normal) ranges. This ability to dynamically self-regulate and ensure balance is maintained is referred to as homeostasis.

Homo- (from Greek, meaning 'same') and *-stasis* (from Greek, meaning 'unchanging state') has been defined concisely by Rutishauser (1999), who suggested that homeostasis is 'the condition of a system when it is able to maintain its essential variables within limits acceptable to its own structure in the face of unexpected disturbances'. On closer examination of this definition, one can see that homeostasis has a number of facets that must be in place if it is to be maintained. Basically these are:

- There must be a system of relationships
- There must be variables, for example concentrations of oxygen, water, sodium, potassium
- The body must be able to monitor for changes in these variables
- The body must have an ability to adjust these variables
- Deficiency or excess of a variable must be damaging in some way to the body
- The body must be able to react to unplanned challenges to these variables.

To illustrate basically how the process of homeostasis operates think for a moment about the challenges that the body faces when a person exercises on a treadmill. Immediately, the muscles used during exercise use more energy than a resting muscle. Exercised muscles need an additional supply of glucose and oxygen in order to produce energy in sufficient quantities to allow the muscle to continue to work. To meet this increase in demand there is an increase in both the heart rate and the respiratory rate, so that the blood can transport more oxygen to the cells. At the same time stored glycogen is converted to glucose and made available to the body, increasing the blood glucose and providing a supply of raw material for energy production. Sweating occurs to assist in keeping the body cool and the person becomes thirsty in response to prompt them to replace the lost water. Each of these changes occurs in order that homeostasis is maintained.

Many of the challenges that the body faces in an exercised state are mirrored at times of acute illness. Illness interrupts the normal homeostatic balance of the body and so the body acts in a manner that seeks to maintain its internal environment. Where illness states differ from exercise is that exercise is self-limiting: when the person is exhausted they will be forced to rest by their body. Where illness is present it can progress and outstrip the body's ability to maintain homeostasis.

Homeostasis and feedback loops

In order to maintain homeostasis, the body must have in place a series of systems that monitor the variables and instigate a response to correct any deviations from the reference ranges. These systems are called feedback loops and can be likened very much to a central heating system commonly found in houses. Figure 2.1 shows how a central heating system is made up of a thermometer (sensor), a heater (effector) and a thermostat (controller). In the central heating system, the controlling thermostat is set to maintain room temperature at a certain level. The sensor or thermometer constantly measures the room temperature to ensure that

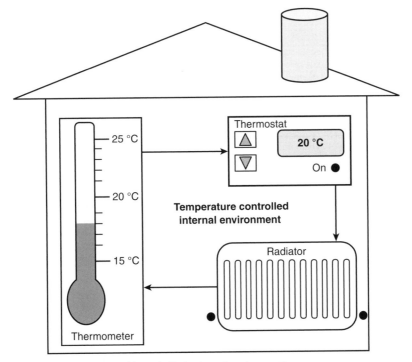

FIGURE 2.1 *Components of a central heating system: negative feedback loop. The thermostat sets the room temperature at 20°C. When the thermometer detects the temperature is below 20°C, the radiator is activated. When the room temperature reaches 20°C, the radiator is deactivated, keeping the room close to 20°C at all times.*

it remains within the set level. If the thermometer senses that the room temperature has fallen, it sends a message to the controller (the thermostat), which in turn sends a message to the effector, the heater, to warm the room. Conversely, once the effector (heater) has performed its role and returned the room temperature to the desired level, the thermometer will sense this and send a message to the controlling thermostat telling it to switch off the heater.

The components and actions that occur in a central heating system are mirrored in the feedback loops that exist within the body to maintain homeostasis. Take for example the regulation of blood glucose outlined in Figure 2.2. You can see that there exist the same components of sensor, controller and effector, and this circuit of components is repeated in all the variables that are under homeostatic control within the body (Box 2.1).

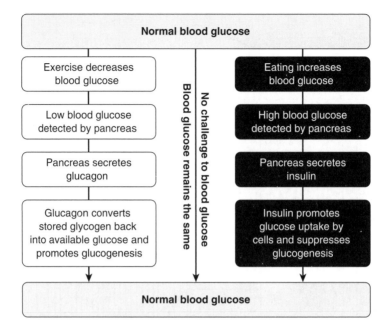

FIGURE 2.2   *Regulation of blood glucose.*

BOX 2.1   Some variables in the body that come under homeostatic control

Reference ranges are shown in brackets

- Temperature (36.3–37.1°C)
- Blood glucose (4–7 mmol/L)
- Blood pressure (110/60–135/85 mmHg)
- Acid–base balance (pH 7.35–7.45)
- Oxygen tension:

  ○ SaO_2 (96–100%)
  ○ PaO_2 (11.89–13.4 kPa; specific range dependent on age)

- Carbon dioxide $PaCO_2$ (4.6–5.9 kPa)
- Electrolytes:

  ○ Na^+ 135–145 mmol/L
  ○ K^+ (serum) 3.5–5.0 mmol/L

From Box 2.1 it is easy to see that the variables that come under homeostatic control are those variables that are commonly assessed as part of observation in the acutely ill. In the clinical setting, therefore, assessing these variables amounts to little more than directly assessing the status of homeostasis. As one would expect, the human body is slightly more complicated than a central heating system and so employs two types of feedback loop to ensure homeostasis is maintained. These are classified as:

- Negative feedback loops
- Positive feedback loops.

Negative feedback loops are responsible for the majority of homeostatic control within the body. They are called negative because they are effectively self-terminating. When the loop has returned the respective variable to an acceptable level, the mechanism switches off. Positive feedback loops are responsible for much fewer responses, but they are of equal importance when considering homeostasis. Positive feedback loops are, as one would expect, the opposite of negative feedback loops. In a positive feedback loop the corrective action occurs, continues and accelerates as a result of continued stimulation; for example uterine contractions during labour are stimulated by the baby's head stretching the cervix. The more the cervix is stretched the more the uterus contracts. Once the baby has been delivered and cervical stretching ceases, uterine contraction stops. The mechanism of blood clotting is another example of a positive feedback loop.

For the body to effect changes in its internal environment, it must constantly monitor the internal environment using sensors. Sensors within the body are basically specialist cells that are sensitised to even the smallest of changes within a given variable. The body is wholly dependent on the effectiveness and accuracy of these sensor sites and should these fail, homeostasis will become disarranged. The sensors are classified according to what they monitor:

- Chemoreceptors: monitor chemical concentrations
- Baroreceptors: monitor pressure
- Osmoreceptors: monitor the osmotic pressure or the amount of water in the body
- Thermoreceptors: monitor the body's temperature.

Various things can cause damage to these sensors. Should this occur, the controller will not receive an accurate picture of what is going on in the body and it follows that the body will then make a control decision to alter its physiology in a way that is potentially damaging to homeostasis. A good example of this occurs in people with essential hypertension. In this case the central nervous system, which controls blood pressure, is slowly reset to accept higher levels of pressure as normal. When this occurs over a long period of time the body fails to recognise this very small upward change in blood pressure and accepts it as normal even though it may be abnormally high. This failure to accurately recognise excessively high pressure will in time lead to organ damage as a result of cells in these organs being compressed and sheared by blood under pressure. In the setting of acute illness, changes occur more abruptly and, depending on the health of the sensors, trigger a rapid response.

Once an abnormality has been detected by a sensor, the body needs to initiate an action to restore homeostasis. The sensor must send a message to the control unit in order to bring about this change. There are two main ways in which the body can achieve this. These are through direct wired nervous control or through chemical messengers such as hormones. Again, if there is a problem with the nerves or an inability to produce hormones, the messages cannot be sent effectively and the controller will not be informed of a challenge to homeostasis. Damage to nerves, for example in neuropathy, or the manipulation of the body's normal responses, say through the use of drugs such as beta-adrenergic blockers, will inhibit the body's ability to understand and react to the messages sent.

The final part of the response to a challenge to homeostasis is to restore the variable to its normal state. This is again achieved via direct nervous control or through hormones. In the acutely ill an understanding of this mechanism is important, as this is often the observable part of acute illness. For example, if a person has a low blood pressure then a combination of nervous signals and chemical messengers will increase the heart rate, cause vasoconstriction, reduce urine output and trigger a sense of thirst. Each of these changes is observable and indicates that that the body is trying hard to maintain homeostasis. The body is able to do this in part due to the presence of extra capacity, for example the ability to breathe deeper or to increase the heart rate. This is called reserve capacity. Problems with the body's ability to self-correct will occur if a person already has an established illness such as chronic obstructive pulmonary disease (COPD). The presence of a pre-existing disease means that the body is already using its reserve capacity which is normally kept for compensating the effects of exercise or acute illness. The existence of pre-existing disease limits a person's ability to compensate for a new disease process and can lead them to become very ill very quickly as homeostasis is disarranged without the ability to correct itself.

Homeostasis and cell energy

Cells of the body carry out many active processes that are related to basic cell activity and the specific specialised function of that given cell type.

More simply, most cells carry out basic functions such as the production of energy and the movement of chemicals in and out of the cell across the cell membrane. Each cell of a specific type, for example nerve cell, cardiac muscle cell or epithelial goblet cell, also carries out a specific function such as the transmission of signals, contraction, or mucus production. Many of the basic and specific functions are classed as active, meaning they require energy to undertake these functions. It follows that if a cell lacks energy it will not be able to fulfil its role and the systems to which the cell belongs will start to fail. Ensuring that cells receive all of the components that they need to generate energy and function correctly is a principal role of homeostasis. Importantly, if homeostasis fails then an increasing number of cells start to fail. This further upsets homeostasis and in turn sets up a cascade of physiological disarrangement which if unopposed will lead to death.

Mostly, cell energy comes in the form of adenosine triphosphate or ATP, a chemical that is manufactured by cells themselves mostly in the mitochondria. The simplest way to think of ATP is as a type of battery that can be used by cells in order to power their activities. A reasonable knowledge of the process that leads to ATP production is needed to understand how the physiological disarrangement which occurs at times of acute illness can lead to energy (ATP) depletion, which directly results in cell dysfunction, injury and death.

To manufacture energy (ATP) the body requires raw materials. The ingredients that are needed for ATP synthesis are carbohydrates, fats and proteins, with carbohydrates providing the majority of the body's energy. In addition to these raw materials, the cells also need an effective transport system and certain other helper chemicals that allow the process to take place most efficiently. Digestive enzymes are needed to break down foods into usable components. Insulin is needed to allow glucose into the cells and oxygen is needed to maximise the amount of energy that is produced. An effective circulation is also required to get the crucial raw materials and helper chemicals to the cell and to remove waste or byproducts of energy production, which can be harmful to the cell when present in excess.

At times of acute illness the energy demands of the body are amplified and at the same time, due to the physiological disarrangement, it is common for a fault to develop in the way that the body produces cell energy. Together, the increased demand for energy and the inability of the body to produce energy place the body in a significantly energy-deficient state. This results in the body having to shut down some of its normal functions in order to conserve energy.

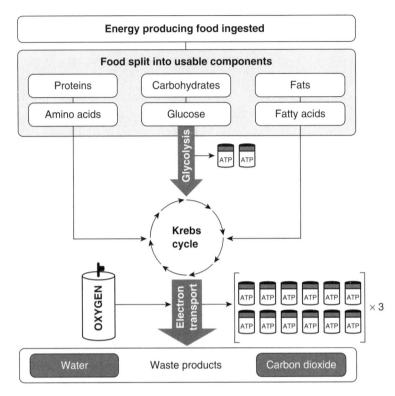

FIGURE 2.3   *The process of cell energy production.*

The human body has adapted to cope with episodes of acute illness for a limited time period in which energy production takes place via an emergency back-up mechanism. Preferentially, in health, the body produces most energy from the breakdown of glucose. This has the benefit of being both efficient and only produces waste products that the healthy body can rid itself of quickly and easily. Converting glucose into ATP is a staged process. An incredibly simple way of explaining this complex process is to consider what enters and exits the chemical reaction at each stage (Figure 2.3). The first step in this process is that a single glucose molecule is split in two and this provides for two ATP batteries. Other chemicals are then further split to produce more ATP. This first part of the process, known as glycolysis, can take place in the absence of oxygen and is referred to as an anaerobic process. While this is helpful in providing cell energy at times of crisis, such as tissue hypoxia, it is a far cry from maximal energy production. For the cell to produce maximal energy from glucose breakdown, oxygen is essential for the second and third stages of the process. Together, this so-called aerobic stage of ATP production contributes most (36 ATP batteries) to the cell's total energy. Thus it is easy to see why oxygen availability to the cells is of paramount importance in maintaining a healthy body.

In situations where glucose is unavailable to the cell due to low blood glucose or an absence of insulin that allows glucose to enter cells, the body derives energy from the breakdown of fats – the so-called fat burning mode. Burning fat is a less attractive process to the body and not all cells are capable of producing energy in this way, although per gram of fuel fat burning actually yields significantly more ATP than the breakdown of glucose. Fat burning can only occur aerobically so there must be oxygen present for the body to generate energy in this way. When glucose is totally unavailable to the cell there is over-production of ketones. Ketones are manufactured mainly in the liver from acetyl coenzyme A, a product of oxidisation of fatty acids (Beckett et al., 2005). Ketones are a useful source of energy for cells such as nerve cells that cannot synthesise energy through the burning of fats, yet the presence of ketones in excess is harmful as they can alter the acidity of the blood and this causes direct injury to cells.

Any discussion of cell energy would be incomplete without at least a mention of the Krebs cycle, which is also known as the citric acid cycle and the tricarboxylic acid cycle. The Krebs cycle is amazingly complex and a detailed explanation is beyond the scope of this text other than to recognise it is important as an aerobic method through which ATP production occurs within the mitochondria. Figure 2.3 shows where the Krebs cycle fits into the process of energy production.

While the chemical reactions that synthesise ATP are very complicated, it is sufficient to recognise that a good supply system gets oxygen and glucose to each cell in the presence of insulin and quickly removes harmful byproducts. The relevance for clinical practice of this is to think that if there is a circulation problem, then raw materials are not being delivered and waste products are not being removed from the cell. If there is an oxygenation problem then cells cannot produce energy most effectively. If there is no insulin then glucose cannot gain access to the cells and be used for energy production. Fat burning will then become the main source of energy with the excessive production of potentially harmful ketones. In short, if the body cannot produce energy, then cells cannot perform their functions and homeostasis is further compromised. If cells are starved of energy for a prolonged period of time then they die and a cascade of homeostatic upset follows. The thinking health professional will consider if their patient has the necessary components for healthy aerobic ATP production and whether these are being delivered in order that the body's cells can function effectively.

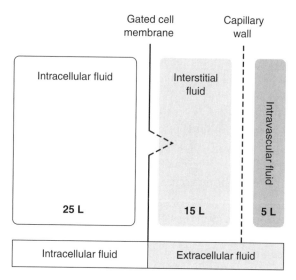

FIGURE 2.4   *Fluid distribution in the body.*

Fluid compartments, fluid shift and osmolarity

Fluid in the body is an exceedingly important transport medium without which important chemicals could not be moved around and exchanged between different parts of the body. Chemicals such as oxygen and glucose are dissolved within body water and if the balance of water in the body is upset, this has far-reaching implications for homeostasis and cell energy production. In the healthy human there are three distinct places where fluid can be found. These places are called fluid compartments.

The three fluid compartments are described as the intracellular space, the interstitial space and the intravascular space. Figure 2.4 provides a schematic view of this concept. The intravascular space is made up of the arteries, capillaries and veins. It is separated from the interstitial space by the walls of the blood vessels. What is immediately obvious from Figure 2.4 is that the fluid contained within the intravascular space (the blood) provides the smallest contribution to the total volume of fluid contained in the body, although this is commonly and erroneously considered to be where the majority of fluid is housed. The majority of fluid is contained within the cells of the body, in the intracellular compartment, which is separated from the interstitial fluid by the semipermeable cell membrane. As the intracellular fluid is a part of a structure it does not have a liquid appearance and as such is essentially hidden. Intracellular fluid is of paramount functional importance as it contributes to the effective transport of chemicals across the cell membrane and the overall functioning of the cell. The interstitial fluid is located between cells and the capillaries. This fluid provides a bridge between the fluid in the intravascular compartment and the intracellular compartment. Chemicals in the blood must pass through the interstitial fluid if they are to reach cells.

The distinct fluid compartments are separated by semipermeable membranes. These are a kind of wall with different gateways and perforations along their length, a bit like checkpoints. These membranes allow fluid and some dissolved chemicals to pass through their walls. Chemicals with large molecular structures are retained in their original compartment and cannot pass through the membrane unless they are invited to do so by a chemical mechanism or as a result of injury, which breaches the integrity of the membrane.

The thin walls of the capillaries separate the intravascular space and the interstitial space, while the cell membrane separates the interstitial and intracellular compartments. To ensure fluid is retained in the correct compartment the body has developed a number of ingenious strategies. These are centred on two factors: the osmotic pressure and the hydrostatic pressure.

The concept of osmotic pressure takes advantage of a solvent potential gradient which is a physical phenomenon that means a solvent (water) moves across a concentration gradient separated by a semipermeable membrane from an area of low concentration to an area of high concentration until equilibrium is established. Figure 2.5 illustrates this diagrammatically. For an example of how osmotic pressure works and helps to keep fluid in the correct space within the body consider the role that albumin or plasma protein plays: albumin is found in comparatively high concentrations in the intravascular space. Albumin has a large molecular structure and as such cannot pass through the walls of the capillaries into the interstitial space unless there is injury to the capillary wall. Thus a comparatively high concentration of albumin exists in the blood. This draws and holds fluid in the intravascular space, hence fluid is partly kept in the intravascular space by the osmotically active presence of albumin. It follows then that if there is a decrease in plasma albumin, excessive fluid can leak into the interstitial space and cause tissue oedema. The principle not only applies to albumin, but also applies to other chemicals in each of the fluid compartments, for example glucose and sodium.

As well as the chemical composition of the body fluid, the physical pressure that exists within a given fluid compartment also plays a part in the movement of fluids between compartments, as does the integrity of the semipermeable membranes of those compartments. If the fluid in one compartment exerts an excessively high pressure on the semipermeable

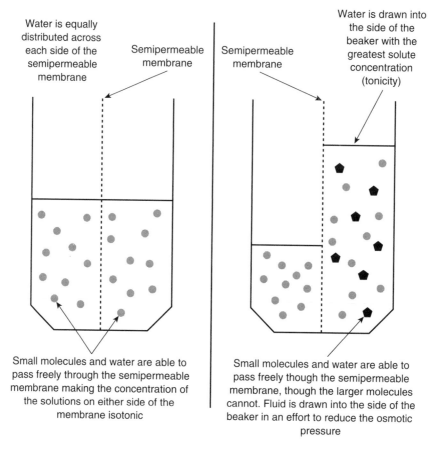

FIGURE 2.5   *Osmosis.*

membrane, then it follows that fluid is more likely to leak out of this compartment no matter how osmotically charged the space may be. An example of this occurs in patients who develop left ventricular failure. This causes a back pressure of blood in the lungs and causes fluid to leak out of the blood into the lungs causing pulmonary oedema. Another classical example of the activity of hydrostatic pressure in fluid shift occurs in older patients who are immobile and develop dependent oedema in the legs. The calf muscle pump, which normally assists in returning blood from the leg against the effect of gravity is made ineffective by immobility. The hydrostatic pressure increases in the intravascular space of the leg due to blood being continually pumped into the leg, but because of the loss of the calf muscle pump, venous return is impaired. This results in a high intravascular pressure, which leads to a leak of fluid into the interstitial space and causes swelling of the limb. The maintenance and shift of fluid between compartments is a balance then between the hydrostatic and osmotic pressures.

In certain disease states, fluid can collect in spaces that do not normally house fluid, such as the peritoneum, pleura and the pericardium. This situation is commonly referred to as third spacing. To illustrate the concept of third spacing, consider how ascites develops. Ascites is the term used to describe a collection of fluid in the peritoneum. The pathogenesis of ascites can be multifactorial, but occurs commonly as a result of impaired blood flow through the liver, which itself has a number of causes such as alcoholic liver disease, infections, malignancy and right-sided heart failure. Blood vessels that drain the intestines (the mesenteric system) empty into the liver in order that digested nutrients can be screened for toxicity by the liver before being forwarded onto the systemic circulation. Anything that inhibits this free flow of blood through the liver causes a back pressure of blood in the mesenteric vessels. This high hydrostatic pressure causes fluid to leak from the intravascular space into the third space, the peritoneum, causing the ascites to develop. Fluid that is displaced because of high hydrostatic pressure, which forces water out of the intravascular space, is referred to as a transudate.

Fluid can also leave the intravascular space and enter a third space because the capillary membrane becomes excessively permeable and allows fluid to leak into the interstitial and third spaces. This type of fluid misdistribution is referred to as an exudate and occurs as a result of inflammation. This phenomenon will be described in more detail later in this chapter (see the section 'The inflammatory response').

Given the importance of fluid within the body as a transport medium and the potential for fluid balance to become disarranged at times of acute illness, it is necessary to consider some clinical terms that assist in understanding a patient's fluid status. Euvolaemia is the term used to describe normal body fluid status. Dehydration describes depletion of whole body fluid. Dehydration can be caused by and will cause hypovolaemia. Hypovolaemia describes a situation where there is low blood volume. It is relatively obvious that bleeding reduces blood volume; what may be less obvious is how hypovolaemia causes dehydration. Hypovolaemia causes dehydration through the process of fluid donation. Fluid donation occurs when fluid is lost from one compartment of the body. This loss of fluid results in the other components giving fluid to the compartment that has become deficient. While this is useful to support the body through short periods of volume depletion, overall it leads to total body dehydration. Fluid can be lost from the body in many ways: it may be the result of blood loss, excessive vomiting and diarrhoea, or an increased urine output, such as in poorly controlled diabetes. Wound exudates may also cause volume depletion.

Hypervolaemia, or fluid overload, rarely occurs spontaneously. When it does occur, it is normally iatrogenic, being the result of over-zealous fluid replacement, although it can occur spontaneously in some conditions such renal (kidney) or heart failure. Both hypovolaemia and hypervolaemia have the potential to cause serious harm and hence, should be monitored for and treated when found.

The maintenance of body fluid is under constant homeostatic control and is managed by fluid intake, urine output and insensible loss in the breath, sweat and faeces. To ensure that the balance of fluid in the body remains constant, both osmo- and baroreceptors are used. The response to fluid loss or fluid gain is mediated by a range of both nervous and hormonal actions. Excessive fluid volume raises the pressure in the blood vessels and cause baroreceptors in the heart to be stretched. This stretching results in a release of the hormone atrial natriuretic peptide (ANP), which in turn makes the kidneys excrete more sodium into the urine taking excess body water with it. The response to fluid loss is a little more complicated and accounts for many of the signs that are seen in the acutely ill. Fluid loss results in a graded chain of events that serve not only to replace fluid lost, but also to maintain perfusion of vital organs while the fluid deficit is being corrected. In the early stages of fluid loss, a reduction in the effective circulating volume is detected by a fall in venous return to the heart. This in turn results in a reduced cardiac output and a slight fall in blood pressure which results in a reduced cerebral and myocardial perfusion. This triggers a chain reaction that aims to restore and maintain perfusion. These reactions are referred to as compensatory mechanisms.

Acid–base disturbance

The human body operates in a slightly alkaline environment with a pH of 7.35–7.45. Any deviation from this narrow range can cause tremendous damage to cells and tissues and so the body has a number of mechanisms to ensure that the acid–base balance of the body is maintained within this narrow range. Simply put these are:

- The ability to excrete carbon dioxide in the lungs
- The ability to excrete acid from the kidneys
- The ability to balance (buffer) the effect of acid and alkaline in the body by balancing their effects against other chemicals.

Many of the chemical reactions that occur within the body produce acids of which the body must rid itself. The process of cell energy production poses a number of challenges to the body's acid–base balance. Carbon dioxide is a byproduct of energy production. It does not exist in the body as a gas but rather is dissolved in body fluids and forms carbonic acid. In health, this carbon dioxide is exhaled from the lungs. If there is a problem with either transporting carbon dioxide to the lungs (a circulatory problem), or exhaling it (a breathing problem), then the pH of the body will fall and the body fluids will become acidic. This gives rise to a condition known as acidosis. As well as the production of carbon dioxide, ATP synthesis can bring about an increase in the amount of acid in the body in two other important ways. When sufficient oxygen is not available to the cell for ATP synthesis then lactic acid is produced, and when there is insufficient glucose available ketone bodies are produced, both of which increase the amount of acid in the blood.

As well as the respiratory system, kidney function plays an important role in maintaining the acid–base balance of the body. A well-perfused kidney excretes excess acid that cannot be exhaled by the lungs. At times of acute illness, a reduction in the effective circulating volume of blood means that the kidneys are not perfused adequately and as a result, they cannot rid the body of the excess acid. The kidneys also govern the amount of bicarbonate in the body, a chemical that is important in buffering the effect of acid and alkaline. A further disturbance of acid–base balance can occur when there is excessive vomiting (a loss of stomach acid) or when there is diarrhoea (with a loss of alkaline mucus from the gut).

Assessment of the acid–base status is undertaken by means of an arterial blood gas test or ABG. This test involves obtaining a sample of arterial blood from the wrist or the groin and quickly analysing it in a special blood gas analyser. The sample is usually obtained using a needle attached to a syringe containing an anticoagulant, although some critically ill patients will have arterial lines inserted and samples can be drawn directly from these. The ABG not only provides information on the pH of the body but also the amount of carbon dioxide ($PaCO_2$), oxygen (PaO_2), bicarbonate and the base excess. The reference ranges for these variables are shown in Box 2.2.

BOX 2.2 Reference ranges for values of variables in an arterial blood gas test

- pH 7.35–7.45 (marker of acute illness severity)
- Partial pressure of carbon dioxide ($PaCO_2$) 4.6–5.9 kPa (measure of ventilation)
- Partial pressure of oxygen (PaO_2) 11.89–13.4 kPa (measure of oxygenation)
- Base excess –2 to +2
- Standard bicarbonate 22–28 mmol/L

Some blood gas analysers provide more information and may detail the lactate, sodium and potassium content of the blood, to name but a few. These values can be used together to identify whether the person has a stable acid–base balance or if there is an acid–base disturbance. There are four principal disturbances of acid–base balance that can occur. These are:

- Respiratory acidosis

  ○ Too much carbon dioxide in the blood (hypoventilation)

- Respiratory alkalosis

  ○ Low carbon dioxide (hyperventilation)

- Metabolic acidosis

  ○ Too much acid in the body (ketones, lactate, ingestion of acid)
  ○ Inability to excrete acid
  ○ Loss of alkaline (diarrhoea)

- Metabolic alkalosis

  ○ Loss of body acids (vomiting).

A mixed acid–base disturbance can also occur if there is a problem with both systems and the body is not able to bring about appropriate compensation.

When an acid–base disturbance occurs the body compensates by adjusting another variable. As there are only two systems involved in acid–base balance, compensation occurs in the counter-system. So, if there is a metabolic acidosis, there will be respiratory compensation and vice versa. Respiratory compensation is rapid, but metabolic compensation takes a while to bring the pH closer to the reference range. Given this time lag, respiratory disturbances of acid–base balance can then be classified as acute (without metabolic compensation) or chronic (with metabolic compensation). Metabolic compensation involves adjusting the amount of bicarbonate that is in the body. Bicarbonate is increased to buffer acid and reduced to buffer alkaline.

The respiratory system compensates for metabolic acidosis by increasing the respiratory rate and depth, so that acidic carbon dioxide is expelled, reducing the $PaCO_2$, and in turn the pH. In metabolic alkalosis, the respiratory effort is reduced, but this is not as powerful a mechanism as is seen in the compensation for metabolic acidosis, for, if it was so, the body would deprive itself of vital oxygen, which is itself alkaline.

Cell insults and death

While highly resilient to insult, human cells are also tremendously fragile and can be damaged in a range of ways that include:

- Deficiency
- Intoxication
- Trauma.

Physically, the human body is a collection of cells that interact in a coordinated fashion. Premature cell death is, in part, death of the human body and if this process is not arrested or it progresses rapidly there is a grave potential for the body as an entity to malfunction and eventually expire. When contemplating cell death in relation to acute illness, it is necessary to consider the events that lead to cell death and put in place measures that prevent these events from occurring. Probably the area where health professionals can do most to avert cell injury and death is in the area of deficiency. In deficiency, cells die because they are not given access to the raw materials needed to produce ATP. Preventing this is concerned with ensuring that homeostasis is maintained. For health professionals this involves performing tests to assess the health of homeostasis and then correcting it artificially if needed.

Cells are also damaged by the presence of toxic substances. Toxins can be produced by the body and not effectively removed, allowing them to build up in concentration to a point where they injure the cell. An excessive level of carbon dioxide (carbonic acid) is an example of how cells can be injured in this way. Alternatively, toxins can be brought in to the body from the outside world. These may be in the form of poisons or drugs, or they may be toxins released by bacteria that have caused an infection. Here the role of the healthcare professional is to assist the body to either neutralise or rid itself of the toxin.

Direct injury to the cell in the form of trauma, burns and radiation can also directly destroy cells. While there is little that health professionals can do to prevent this, once it has already occurred there is much that can be done to prevent subsequent infection and further tissue loss.

The inflammatory response

Once cells die, they send out chemical messages that are recognised by the body as a kind of SOS signal and the body mounts an inflammatory response which is targeted at disposing of the cell debris and removing infection that may be present. To understand the inflammatory response think back to a time when you have had a spot or boil. These common skin infections classically cause pain, swelling, localised heat and reddening of the skin. These are signs of inflammation and occur any time cells are destroyed and not just at times of infection. They occur as the body attempts to put in place a system of measures that restore homeostasis and limit the effects of the injury or insult.

Figure 2.6 shows in a simple manner what happens during the inflammatory process. Pro-inflammatory cytokines are initially released into the body. This causes the semipermeable membrane of the capillary bed to become more permeable than usual, allowing more fluid to leak into the tissues, causing local swelling. Specialist white blood cells known as neutrophils and macrophages are drawn to the site of the injury following the chemical messages. These then start the process of phagocytosis (eating dead tissue and bacteria) in order to cleanse the area. Once the debris has been removed, new tissue can regrow if the tissue type affected is capable of this. Where the tissue is not capable of regrowth, the necrotic tissue will be removed and scar tissue will form. This scarring can cause significant dysfunction to organs.

Compensatory mechanisms: putting it all together

When the body faces a particular challenge, say loss of fluid, the body makes an effort to compensate for this to maintain homeostasis. These compensatory mechanisms are often the visible part of acute illness and the pointers that alert health professionals to the presence of an acute

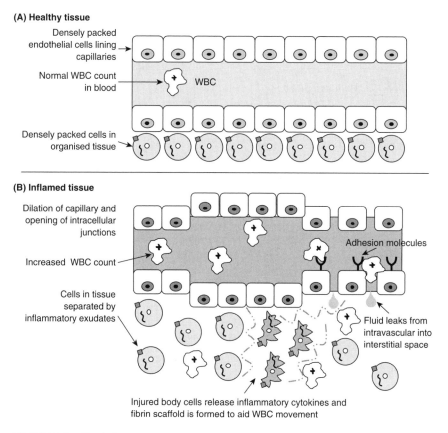

(A) Healthy tissue

Densely packed endothelial cells lining capillaries

Normal WBC count in blood — WBC

Densely packed cells in organised tissue

(B) Inflamed tissue

Dilation of capillary and opening of intracellular junctions

Increased WBC count

Adhesion molecules

Cells in tissue separated by inflammatory exudates

Fluid leaks from intravascular into interstitial space

Injured body cells release inflammatory cytokines and fibrin scaffold is formed to aid WBC movement

FIGURE 2.6   *The inflammatory response. WBC, white blood cell.*

illness. Unfortunately, compensation in an otherwise healthy individual can mask serious disease until such a stage that the person can no longer compensate and the person becomes seriously unwell in a very short period of time. Sadly this is a common occurrence in children, who have a tremendous reserve capacity, allowing catastrophic organ damage to occur before they decompensate. It is essential that health-care professionals can recognise the signs that a compensatory mechanism has been activated as well as knowing the factors that will limit a person's ability to mount a full compensatory response. This is discussed in Chapter 3.

To understand how compensation works, take, for example, a person who has lost fluid because of excessive vomiting. The person is said to be hypovolaemic. Due to the reduced circulating volume of fluid, the body compensates by moving the fluid that it has remaining more quickly

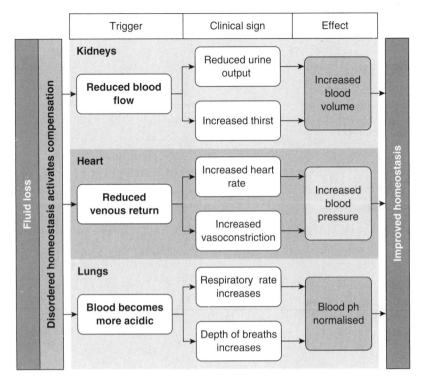

FIGURE 2.7   *Summary of activated compensatory mechanisms.*

around the system in order that it can continue to effectively perfuse the tissues. This is manifested as tachycardia, one of the signs of hypovolae-mia. Additionally, the person's respiratory rate will increase as there is a need to oxygenate the blood more rapidly. The production of urine will decrease in order that the body retains volume. Fluid will be drawn into the intravascular compartment from the interstitial space to compensate for the intravascular loss and the blood vessels will contract. The result of this is that a normal or slightly elevated blood pressure will be main-tained. If the fluid loss is not arrested or is particularly rapid in its occur-rence, then the body will come to the limits of compensation and the disease process will outstrip the body's ability to compensate. This is termed decompensation and during this phase cell death occurs and eventually the person will die if no intervention is provided. Box 2.3 summarises the clinical findings that indicate a body is compensating physiological disarrangement and Figure 2.7 illustrates the relationships in the compensatory mechanism.

BOX 2.3 Clinical findings in compensation

Early signs that indicate compensatory mechanisms are activated

- Change in pulse pressure
- Tachypnoea
- Reduced urine output
- Increased capillary refill time
- Slight increase in heart rate

Factors that limit a person's ability to compensate for illness

- Pre-existing illness
- Beta-blocking drugs
- Angiotensin-converting enzyme inhibitor drugs

The development of disease

The body's ability to tolerate significant insult, then adjust and repair without conscious thought, is a fascinating attribute. Occasionally, the mechanisms that are responsible for ensuring the maintenance of homeostasis either fail, become overwhelmed or react over-zealously. When this occurs, in isolation or in combination, there is significant potential for cellular injury to occur.

Having defined homeostasis it is necessary, yet relatively simple, to define what is meant by a disease or illness state. On the simplest of levels, disease can be defined as a failure of homeostasis. While this will to some degree explain what disease is, it does little to explain what caused the homeostatic mechanisms to fail and the body to become unbalanced. To adequately explain this, it is necessary to introduce a further concept, the aetiology of disease. Aetiology is the cause of a disease and there are many examples of different aetiologies, but what is common to them all is that they have the potential to cause damage to cellular structures and as a result cell injury, dysfunction or premature cell death.

Having established that aetiology is the cause of the disease, there is one final part of the picture that needs to be included before a full understanding can be achieved. This final component is pathogenesis, which is the pathological mechanism which results in clinically evident disease (Lakhanin et al., 2003). Understanding pathogenesis is probably as important as understanding homeostasis. This is true because if one understands how a disease is caused, you can understand how it can be prevented or its effects mitigated. A second reason for understanding pathogenesis is that not all aetiological factors will cause disease in all patients and that often a set of factors need to come together in order for a disease to manifest itself. To illustrate the stages of disease development, consider the example in Box 2.4.

BOX 2.4   An example of homeostatic disarrangement

Mrs Jones is a 64-year-old woman living in a nursing home. Three years ago she had a significant stroke, which left her with significant disability and an inability to speak. At the time of her stroke, she was found to have type 2 diabetes mellitus and hypertension. Both of these factors were thought to have contributed to her developing a stroke. Mrs Jones's diabetes is normally controlled using diet alone. Over the last week, she developed symptoms that were suggestive of a chest infection and was started on antibiotic therapy by her general practice. Despite this, she has become increasingly drowsy over the last week and has required acute hospital admission despite the apparent resolution of her chest infection.

Questions

1 What disease process do you think has developed in Mrs Jones?
2 Which variables that are under homeostatic control are likely to be disarranged?
3 What tests do you think Mrs Jones requires?
4 Can you suggest a management plan for her?

Answer

The diagnosis that Mrs Jones received was hyperosmolar non-ketotic state (HONK). This is a condition that develops mainly in people with type 2 diabetes, particularly when patients are suffering from a concurrent illness or infection. In Mrs Jones's case, the infection caused her body to become under stress. At times of stress, the body releases hormones to help it to deal with the problem. These hormones, principally adrenaline and cortisol, have an opposing effect to insulin and thus cause the blood sugar to rise. In the healthy individual, additional insulin would be released and the blood glucose would be returned to normal levels. In the person with diabetes, the already damaged pancreatic islets cells cannot produce sufficient additional insulin to compensate for the increase in blood glucose and the blood glucose level becomes elevated far above the normal range. The more serious the infection, the more stress hormones will be released and the higher the blood glucose will become.

> The rise in the blood glucose causes the body to react by excreting glucose in the urine. This takes water with it and depletes the intravascular space. The blood (intravascular space) is now highly concentrated and this causes water from other parts of the body to be drawn into the intravascular space causing total body dehydration. The person would become thirsty, but in patients such as Mrs Jones who is unable to communicate this feeling, the blood glucose continues to rise and the dehydration will be worsened. This has a sequel of making the blood more susceptible to clotting and the person experiences a stroke or myocardial infarction. Homeostatic management will involve finding and treating the infective cause (antibiotics), correcting the blood glucose (insulin infusion) and replacing lost fluid and electrolytes (IV fluid ± potassium).

The case study in Box 2.4 illustrates how people can develop an acute condition on top of a chronic disease, the so-called acute-on-chronic phenomenon. In Mrs Jones, the acute complication is a direct result of the long-standing illness and could not have occurred without its presence. It is also possible to see that the acute condition HONK is a clear example of a cascade of homeostatic disarrangements affecting a significant number of variables within the body that are normally tightly controlled in health. Furthermore, the case study illustrates how the stress response, a mechanism intended to assist the body to manage stressful or dangerous situations, can actually contribute to the development of an illness state.

Overexcited and exhausted physiological responses

Occasionally, the mechanisms that the body has in place to solve problems and compensate for acute illness turn against the body and become illness states in their own right. These conditions are often serious and are considered to be pre-terminal events. There are two important conditions, the pathogenesis of which is logical when one understands the basis of how the body reacts to insult: systemic inflammatory response syndrome (SIRS) and disseminated intravascular coagulopathy (DIC) are both examples of when the body is overwhelmed by widespread insult and reaches the limits of its ability to cope.

In SIRS the widespread inflammation within the body leads to an opening of the multiple capillary beds, allowing fluid to leak out from the intravascular space into the interstitial space across the whole body. This has the consequence of depleting the intravascular space and dropping the blood pressure, reducing organ perfusion. Intravenous fluid replacement simply leaks into the interstitial space making the condition difficult to treat without the addition of vasoactive drugs.

In DIC the pro-inflammatory chemicals that initiate coagulation at the site of injury are released as normal. DIC occurs when illness is widespread and coagulation occurs throughout the body. Platelets, an important part of the coagulation cascade, are only available in a limited supply, and when illness is widespread the supply of platelets is quickly exhausted. The clinical consequence of this is the formation of multiple small clots in the blood. This makes the blood into a kind of slurry, the circulation of which is near impossible. With an absence of platelets, the blood can no longer clot and bleeding occurs from multiple sites and the person can die from infarction or blood loss if the DIC cannot be corrected.

Acute respiratory distress syndrome

A final condition that warrants mention is acute respiratory distress syndrome (ARDS). ARDS has a number of synonyms from adult respiratory distress syndrome to acute lung injury. No matter what the condition is termed, it is a serious pulmonary complication of acute illness. It can arise as a result of direct injury to the lung or via a significant insult to the body elsewhere. Sepsis, major trauma, massive blood transfusion and pneumonia are all common causes. Patients with ARDS will experience pulmonary oedema with hypoxia and respiratory failure. This may resolve or progress to fibrosis (scarring) of the lungs. ARDS has a high mortality rate and those who do survive are often left with residual disability in the form of breathlessness.

Conclusion

The emphasis of this chapter has been on stressing the importance of homeostasis. When people become acutely ill, homeostatic processes fail and it is the abnormal findings of a given variable that indicate to health professionals that a person is unwell. The role of the health professional is to recognise that the person is unwell and initiate treatment. Treatment for these patients involves homeostatic resuscitation, by restoring the variable to the reference range. It involves identifying an abnormal variable within the body, such as the blood pressure and then setting a target range for it to be maintained within through treatment, for example titration of intravenous fluids to keep the systolic blood pressure at 90 mmHg. Using goal-directed therapy (Chapter 1) means that not only are abnormal findings recognised and treatment given, but most importantly a test is done to confirm that the treatment has been effective and that homeostasis has been restored, albeit artificially, until the body is able to resume this action for itself.

Using goal–directed therapy ensures that patients are constantly monitored in the light of their response to treatment. If the prescribed plan of care is not sufficient to maintain the person, then care can be, if needed, escalated to provide maximal homeostatic support and the best possible outcome for the patient.

 Key learning points

- The human body is an amazingly complex entity.
- The body strives to protect the internal environment and maintain homeostatic balance within narrow limits.
- Injury or insult to one part of the body can bring about compensation in other parts of the body.
- Compensation can mask severe illness, if not looked for carefully.
- Cells can tolerate significant insult before they are irreversibly damaged, leading to cell death.
- This makes cell death a potentially preventable condition if early recognition and intervention is provided.
- Cell death initiates an inflammatory response.
- Widespread inflammation can result in disseminated intravascular coagulopathy or systemic inflammatory response syndrome, which can quickly result in death.
- Use early goal-directed therapies to ensure that homeostasis is maintained.
- In order to achieve this, health professionals must understand the physiological response to acute illness so that its presence can be quickly identified and managed.

Self-assessment questions

1 Homeostasis can be defined as:

   A   The inability of the body to maintain its own environment
   B   The condition of a system when it is able to maintain its essential variables within limits acceptable to its own structure in the face of unexpected disturbances

(Continued)

(Continued)

C   The balance of oxygen and fluid within the body
D   The process through which cell energy is produced
E   The process that prevents inflammation in healthy tissues

2   Pathogenesis is the term used to describe:

A   The study of disease
B   The mechanism that converts aetiology into disease
C   The way that the body maintains homeostasis
D   A predisposition towards developing a disease
E   The point at which a disease process becomes clinically evident

3   Which one of the following is not required for most effective production of ATP?

A   Glucose
B   Oxygen
C   Insulin
D   Albumin
E   Mitochondria

4   Which one of the following is an example of an aetiology?

A   Tachycardia
B   Vomiting
C   Abdominal pain
D   Norwalk virus
E   Dehydration

5   The fluid compartments contained in the body are correctly classified as:

A   Intracellular, intravenous, intrathecal
B   First space, second space, third space
C   Intravascular, interstitial, intracellular
D   Arterial, capillary, venous
E   Intercellular

6   Decompensation

A   Occurs when a person has died and the tissue is destroyed
B   Represents at the start of a disease process causing physiological disarrangement, but no clinically overt disease
C   Is the point at which the disease outstrips the body's ability to self-repair
D   Is the ability of the body to react to a disease process and limit the effect that it has on the body
E   Is the sharing of fluid between compartments after a loss of fluid is sustained from one compartment

7   Anaerobic respiration:

   A   Occurs in the absence of adequate oxygen supplies
   B   Is inefficient in producing ATP
   C   Results in the production of harmful lactic acid
   D   Is used only in physiological emergencies where other methods for
       ATP synthesis are not available
   E   All of the above

8   In the breakdown of fats to produce energy, which of the following can be
    used as an emergency form of energy by some cells?

   A   Carbon dioxide
   B   Lactic acid
   C   Ketones
   D   Water
   E   Triglycerides

9   Goal-directed therapy is:

   A   Of no benefit outside of the critical care area
   B   Time consuming, leading to extra paperwork and detracting from
       patient care
   C   Helpful as it means that homeostasis is maintained
   D   Can only be delivered by specially trained individuals
   E   Occurs at the expense of holistic care

10 Which one of the following is not a part of the compensatory mechanism
    in significant fluid loss?

   A   Tachycardia
   B   Tachypnoea
   C   Low blood pressure
   D   Reduced urine output
   E   Thirst

Answers

1B, 2B, 3D, 4D, 5C, 6C, 7E, 8C, 9C, 10C.

Further reading

Lakhanin, S., Dilly, D., Finlayson, C. and Dogan, A. (2003) *Basic Pathology: An
   Introduction to the Mechanisms of Disease*. London: Hodder Arnold.
This text expands on some of the pathological concepts such as the inflammatory
response that lead to the development of disease. It also contains chapters on specific
diseases which are relevant to those caring for the acutely ill.

Popcock, G. and Richards, C.D. (2006) *Human Physiology: The Basis of Medicine*, 3rd edn. Oxford: Oxford University Press.
This is a detailed physiology text that is principally aimed at the medical student, yet its approach to the subject is both complete and understandable for those willing to invest a little effort.

Tortora, G.J. and Nielsen, M.T. (2009) *Principles of Human Anatomy*, 11th edn. Oxford: John Wiley & Sons.
This is a classic anatomy text that will help those interested to develop a more detailed view of how the body is structured.

3

Patient stability assessment

Chapter aims

By the end of this chapter you should be able to:

- Describe a systematic approach to assessing those at risk of becoming acutely ill
- Link clinical findings to an understanding of the changing physiology that occurs during episodes of acute illness
- Successfully identify those who have become acutely ill and require interventions

Chapter 1 established that the early recognition of and intervention in those who are acutely ill leads to dramatically improved outcomes. Yet too often the opportunity of early intervention is missed as patients are not recognised as being acutely ill until such a point that they deteriorate to the extent where their illness becomes obvious even to the untrained observer. To address this issue and improve patient outcomes, health professionals working with people at risk of becoming acutely ill must adopt a manner of working that is effective in quickly identifying patients at risk with a high degree of specificity and sensitivity. In order to achieve this, two factors must be brought together. Firstly, a minimum set of information about the patient's condition must be gathered as a base for decision making. Secondly, health professionals must hold sufficient knowledge of the physiology of acute illness that allows them to deduce what is happening with the patient and draw conclusions about their stability. If either one of these components is absent patients will be placed at risk of unrecognised deterioration.

Gathering the needed data through the performance of basic physiological observations of a patient's vital signs is a skill that can be quickly learnt, yet is often performed poorly or incompletely. This chapter aims to reignite interest in the importance of rigorous patient assessment and provides a systematic framework of assessment that can be used in practice to identify those who are acutely ill. Essentially, this includes screening patients for signs of acute illness or physiological disarrangement. It focuses on getting the basic components of assessment right and initiating a response when needed. Accordingly this chapter is divided into two parts: the first overviews a model of assessment that can be used, with the second part describing how to perform and interpret the findings of patient assessment.

Part one: a framework for assessing patients

Changing the mindset

Performing observations of a patient's vital signs is all too commonly seen as little more than a chore that must be completed and documented ritualistically, rather than an important assessment of the patient's condition. While all members of the healthcare team have a contribution to make, there needs to be an appreciation of the scope of practice of each individual member. Interpretation of a patient's vital signs can be complex for the novice and junior members of the team and they should not be expected to undertake this task alone without the support of more senior colleagues. The reasons for this are outlined below.

One conceptual problem with observations is the term itself, as it implies that all that is required is a passive observation of the patient's condition and ritualistic charting of the information. A preferred term is patient stability assessment (PSA). This conjures ideas of not only the collection of information, but also the need to make judgements about this information and decide on a plan for further assessment and management.

The plural nature of the word 'observations' implies that the parameters observed (e.g. pulse and blood pressure) are useful in isolation. This creates the second problem with the term 'observations'. Indeed much information can be gathered about a patient from assessment of their pulse, but this provides only limited information about the patient's overall stability. In order to make a complete patient stability assessment, a full set of vital signs needs to be recorded to be able to reach a defensible decision. There may well be situations where the assessment of individual parameters is useful in other areas of healthcare, such as the monitoring of blood pressure in a person being treated for hypertension. However, these are outside the scope of this chapter.

The third problem is overreliance on perceived normal values for each parameter measured. Accepting without questioning that a patient's vital signs are in the normal ranges is a false reassurance. While there are ranges of values which are considered normal, these must be interpreted in the light of the condition of the individual patient. There must also be an appreciation of how the observations have changed over time and this leads on to the fourth problem with observations. This fourth problem is concerned with undertaking a single set of observations without follow-up to look for any changes that have occurred within the perceived normal values. Again this can lead to a false reassurance of patient stability.

The fifth and final problem with observations relates to the quality of technique that is used to gather data about the patient. The accuracy and precision of the data gathered are directly related to the quality of the technique used to collect it. A poor-quality technique can lead to spurious results which will cloud the decision-making process and impact on patient care. It is thus essential that the correct technique is used each time a measurement is made and the limits of that assessment are understood by the person making the measurement. Given these problems, you are urged to abandon the term 'observations' in favour of the concept of PSA, as this better reflects the process that must be undertaken if those who are acutely ill are to be identified and managed appropriately in a timely fashion.

Establishing a minimum dataset for patient stability assessment

In order to make any valid and reliable assessment of a patient's condition one requires sufficient and accurate information on which to base the decision. This should be thought of as the minimum dataset, or the minimum amount of information that is needed in order to make a reliable assessment of a patient's condition. It is essential to recognise that a patient's condition cannot be accurately assessed by looking at isolated parameters such as blood pressure and pulse rate alone. All of the vital signs are needed to make a complete and correct PSA. You must never try to circumvent this process by taking shortcuts and neglecting to collect all the required information as this is likely to lead to suboptimal care for patients and could form the basis of a negligence claim.

The information needed to make a PSA can be divided into:

- **End of bed assessment**: all patients continually.
- **Screening tests**: all patients when planned or if a deterioration is suspected
- **Trend assessment**: after each set of screening tests
- **Comprehensive additional tests**: when indicated.

End of bed assessment

The process of assessment includes making an initial check of the patient from the 'end of the bed'. This serves to give you a crude picture of how ill you think the person is. While a little subjective, being able to make a rapid yet rough assessment of the severity of a patient's illness is a good skill to have. It enables you to quickly assess all patients continually and to decide if further stability assessment is appropriate or if resuscitation should be initiated. Box 3.1 outlines points that you should consider when undertaking an end of bed assessment.

BOX 3.1   Points to consider in an end of bed assessment

- Is the person conscious or unconscious?
- Are they **a**lert or responsive to **v**oice or **p**ain or are they **u**nresponsive (AVPU)?
- What is their demeanour? Confused, agitated, in pain, quiet, guarded?
- What is their skin colour? Pale, cyanosed, reddish, obvious rash?
- How much effort is going into breathing? Little, normal, laboured?
- Does the person appear to be in pain or in distress?
- Objects around the person – vomit bowls, intravenous infusions, oxygen, nebulisers, etc., to give clues.

Screening tests

The screening tests needed to make a decision about patient stability are those that would have been traditionally considered standard nursing observations, with some possible additions. The results of these tests provide the bulk of information needed to make a PSA. The tests needed to collect the minimum dataset are listed in Box 3.2.

BOX 3.2   Minimum dataset needed to make a PSA

- Conscious level
- Capillary refill
- Respiratory: rate, rhythm, symmetry

- Pulse: rate, rhythm, volume
- Blood pressure: systolic, diastolic, mean arterial, pulse pressure
- Oxygen saturation
- Temperature: core, extremities
- Fluid balance: fluid intake, urine output, vomiting, other outputs
- Pain

The purpose of the screening tests is to directly examine a person's physiological state in order to identify if a compensatory mechanism has been activated. While each variable – pulse, respiratory rate, etc. – is important in its own right, more subtle changes in a patient's condition can be identified by looking at the sum of what all the observations are telling you, hence the need to undertake all of the observations at each assessment.

To illustrate this, consider the case of a 19-year-old athletic man admitted to your care with abdominal pain of unknown cause. His screening observations are: pulse 88 beats per minute, regular, thready; blood pressure 132/64 mmHg; pulse pressure 68 mmHg; mean arterial pressure 86 mmHg; respiratory rate 18 beats per minute, normal depth, no accessory muscle use; equal chest expansion; SaO_2 96% on room air; conscious level alert; and not passed urine in the last four hours despite intravenous fluids. The majority of these observations in isolation could be considered normal; in fact the pulse, respiratory rate, SaO_2, consciousness level, blood pressure all score 0 on commonly used early warning scoring (EWS) systems. The urine output is the only parameter that is outside its reference range, and in isolation could be little cause for concern, especially if the patient reports this to be usual for him. However, when one considers the wide pulse pressure of 68 mmHg, suggesting possible early vasoconstriction, and an absence of urine output with a pulse and respiratory rate heading towards the upper level of normal in an athletic man, one should be aware of the possibility of volume depletion. Using capillary refill and assessing the skin temperature will further confirm this and add additional information about the patient's condition. While pain may be the cause of these changes, it is worth performing serial assessments of this patient to identify its true cause.

Trend assessment
Trends or changes in a person's screening tests are of equal importance to the actual values that are obtained. Changes in a parameter's value between assessment periods can help to identify early deterioration in a patient before it becomes obvious even to the untrained observer. Assessment of trends is

necessary as the range of what would be considered normal (the reference range) can be quite wide. Take for example the reference range for pulse rate, which is accepted as being 61–99 beats per minute – there are 38 findings that would be considered normal. While each of these individual values may be acceptable in isolation, a change in pulse rate from 61 beats per minute at the start of the day to 90 beats per minute at the end of the day is a significant shift and could be an early warning of acute illness.

Changes over time can be quite subtle, say 5 mmHg in blood pressure or 5 beats per minute in the pulse rate. If you assess the patient every two hours and see an increase in heart rate of 5 beats per minute compared with the previous result then there is temptation to see this as a normal variation. Examination of results must extend beyond the previous result and consider all the results to reveal a gradual change over a period of hours or days. For example, over a ten-hour period the person's pulse could have changed from its initial reading by 30 beats per minute, yet still remain in the reference range. This change is noteworthy and warrants further investigation as to its cause, despite being possibly considered as a normal pulse rate.

Comprehensive and additional testing

In addition to the minimum dataset screening tests that have been described above, there will be times when a more focused and detailed assessment is required. Some patients will require specific monitoring of parameters that have not already been described here. For example, patients with diabetes mellitus may require their blood glucose levels monitoring and patients with asthma may require peak expiratory flow rate assessment. The exact tests to be performed and frequency of assessment should be recorded as a part of the patient's care plan. Additional testing seeks to identify exactly what the cause of a problem is in order that specific management can be provided. Consider, for example, that you discover a patient to have developed a tachycardia of 144 beats per minute. They have a blood pressure in a range usual for them, with a slight increase in respiratory rate since their last assessment. In this circumstance a 12-lead electrocardiogram would be a helpful test to assist in classifying the tachycardia.

Making the patient stability assessment

Once the above information has been collected, it can be used to make the PSA. The PSA should be seen as an assessment that is informed by the information gathered. Failure to collect any of the minimum dataset effectively means that the PSA cannot be made. Making the PSA requires the interpretation of the results of the screening and any additional tests that were performed. Decision making for a PSA commands the application of knowledge about the physiology of acute illness as one is trying to identify if any signs of compensation are evident.

The interpretation of patient data must also be done in the light of any concurrent treatment that the patient is receiving as this will impact on the PSA. For example, if a patient with pneumonia has an oxygen saturation of 92% on room air, this is a less worrying finding than if they have a saturation of 93% while breathing a high concentration of oxygen (80%) through a non-rebreathe mask. Remember that beta-blockers and drugs that interfere with the renin–angiotensin–aldosterone system will also have an impact on a person's ability to initiate a compensatory mechanism and therefore they will not exhibit classic signs of compensation and could lead you to falsely believe the patient to be well, when in truth they could be acutely ill. When a drug that a patient is taking can affect the person's ability to compensate this should be flagged on the assessment chart. While making a PSA, try to answer the 12 questions in Box 3.3. The purpose of these questions is to ensure that you use the information gathered and relate them to the patient and to the physiological changes that occur in the acutely ill.

BOX 3.3 Questions to ask yourself when making a PSA

Airway

1 Is this person's airway clear or is it compromised/at risk?

Breathing

2 Is this person ventilating well (moving air)?
3 Is this person oxygenating well (absorbing oxygen from the air moved)?

Circulation

4 Does this person have an adequate blood volume?
5 Is the blood volume circulating effectively?

Disability

6 Is there normal neurological function?

Decide

7 Is there any reason why this person would have atypical findings?
8 Has there been a change in this person since the last assessment?
9 Is this patient stable or showing signs of compensating?
10 Do you need any more information to truly make this judgement?
11 What are this person's problems?
12 What is my plan for assessment and management?

TABLE 3.1   *Example of an early warning score (EWS) (Prytherch et al., 2010)*

Score	3	2	1	0	1	2	3
Pulse (beats per minute)		<40	41–50	51–90	91–110	111–130	>131
Breathing rate (breaths per minute)	<8		9–11	12–20		21–24	>25
Temperature ($°C$)	<35.0		35.1–36.0	36.1–38.0	38.1–39.0	>39.1	
Systolic blood pressure (mmHg)	<90	91–100	101–110	111–249	>250		
Oxygen saturation (%)	<91	92–93	94–95	>96			
Inspired oxygen				Air			Any O_2
CNS use (AVPU scale)				Alert (A)			Voice (V) Pain (P) Unresponsive (U)

Drawing conclusions about a patient's stability can be a difficult task to perform and calculation of an EWS (Table 3.1) can in some cases help to establish if a person has observations that, when brought together, indicate that the person is in the early stages of becoming acutely ill. You must recognise however that EWS systems are decision-support tools to assist you in making a decision and cannot be used without an understanding of the physiological changes that take place during an episode of acute illness. Most EWS systems work by assigning a score to each of the variables that are commonly assessed when assessing patients. The score is assigned according to how far away from normal the value is. The score is then totalled to give the final EWS. Predetermined trigger points are set and if the patient's score exceeds one of these points, then it is an indication to act.

Caution is needed when using EWS systems as not all of them are well validated. Different scoring systems base the score on different parameters and some also weight the values of the parameters differently. Thresholds for actions may also vary between scoring systems and this may cause confusion if different systems are in use in different areas of the hospital. Many EWS systems work on the principle that the patient had normal parameters at the start of the episode of illness, and as a result do not take into account individual variability such as patients with pre-existing hypertension. A final caution with the use of EWS systems is concerned with their inability to take into account other treatments that a patient may be taking that either impact on the body's ability to compensate for illness or support the body to cope with illness. The sample score provided in Table 3.1 and the associated work by Prytherch et al. (2010) has gone a good way to combat some these traditional problems associated with EWS systems.

Action planning

Once the PSA has been undertaken and decisions made, it is important to devise a plan of care which is appropriate to the needs of the patient. This process could involve deciding that a patient is stable and can be reassessed in four hours, or involve recognising that there is an abnormality and further assessment or intervention is required immediately. One of the most difficult decisions to make is that a person is stable and requires no further investigation and management at this time, as this requires a wide range of criteria to be fulfilled and thus, one should always exercise caution when drawing this conclusion.

There will be circumstances where, in the main, the parameters of the minimum dataset are within the normal ranges, but are close to the limits of normal, or there is one parameter that is not totally acceptable, yet not critical. In these circumstances, the appropriate decision is to consider how frequently you need to perform a PSA on a patient. Each time you assess the patient, plan when the next PSA should be undertaken. Do not rigidly stick to the use of four-hourly observations as it does not reflect the dynamic needs of patients; increase the frequency of PSAs when you see a need to do so. As a minimum, the National Institute for Health and Clinical Excellence (NICE, 2007) recommends that patients in hospital are assessed every 12 hours. If at any point you identify a finding that is potentially life-threatening, such as profound bradycardia, you should stop the screening and summon help and provide any needed treatment.

Documenting your findings

Documenting the result of the screening tests and the PSA is very important, as it not only allows for the identification of trends in a patient's condition, but it also demonstrates that appropriate assessments were made and the correct action taken. Most healthcare settings have a standard form for recording all the information which is needed to undertake a full screening of a patient's stability. It is important that you check that there is space to record all the information you require in a way that allows that information to be easily interpreted. Each hospital will have a policy on documentation and you should familiarise yourself with this. It is worth noting that in addition to recording the patient's assessments on the monitoring chart, it is also important to document in the patient's notes any abnormalities and the action taken to correct these, along with the patient's response. A summary statement in the notes at both the start and end of your period of duty is worthwhile.

Part two: performing patient stability assessments and understanding the significance

In part one of this chapter, a model for PSA was outlined. In this second part, details of how to perform each of the screening tests will be provided. When performing screening tests, it is helpful to follow a standard approach each and every time you perform them. This way you will become familiar with the tests that need to be performed and you will appear more confident and be less likely to miss out any tests. Adopting a standard approach will also assist you by allowing you to think more about the findings of the tests, rather than what test you need to undertake next. Finally, linking the tests in a logical order makes you appear more organised and professional.

As with all patient interactions, it is important that the patient is kept informed and gives consent for you to perform these tests. Ensure that you follow infection control procedures and decontaminate your hands before and after patient contact. Consider that for some patients who feel ill or who are in pain, repeated assessments of their condition may become burdensome and you should do all you can to minimise this and not exacerbate any pain that the patient may have.

The quality of technique used to gather information about patients is tremendously important as incorrect information will lead to an incorrect assessment of patient stability. While the tests used in screening for acute illness are quite basic, many people are tempted to take shortcuts or fail to fully appreciate all of the findings possible. It is for this reason that the salient points in how to perform these tests are outlined here.

Level of consciousness

A patient's level of consciousness is one of the first things that you should assess and is something that you can assess quite quickly. While it is likely to be obvious that a patient is unconscious, more subtle changes in a patient's level of consciousness may be more difficult to appreciate. There are many factors that can alter a person's level of consciousness, making it an important marker of acute illness. Some of the causes of an altered level of consciousness will be as a result of a systemic disease process such as hypoxia or toxicity. Indeed, an important systemic cause of an altered level of consciousness is low blood glucose (hypoglycaemia) and any patient with an altered level of consciousness should have their blood glucose measured as a matter of routine. Others causes of an altered level of consciousness will relate to a more local problem with the functioning of the brain such as an acute rise in intracranial pressure.

In some patients with long-term health conditions who may have previously had a stroke or have developed dementia, assessing the person's level of consciousness can be quite challenging and it may well be quite unreliable. Here, the advice of someone known to the patient can be invaluable in determining the person's usual state of consciousness.

To assess the patient's level of consciousness the AVPU scale is used. As mentioned in part one of this chapter, 'A' signifies that the patient is alert; 'V' indicates that the patient only responds to verbal stimuli; 'P' that the patient responds to only painful stimuli; and 'U' indicates that the patient is unresponsive. To use the AVPU scale, look at your patient: if they are sitting up and talking to others, then they can be classified as alert. If the patient is quiet and not showing any interaction with their environment, but responds to you calling their name or asking if they are okay, then they can be classified as responding to verbal stimuli. When assessing response to voice, care needs to be used in order to discriminate between a patient who is resting and one who requires continued verbal stimulation to maintain concentration. If there is no response to verbal stimuli it is necessary to test a patient's response to a painful stimulus. Pain is a protective sensation and in health the body responds to pain in a way to protect itself from injury. It is therefore normal for a patient who experiences pain to respond in some purposeful way and try to remove the cause of pain. This is known as 'localising to pain'. As well as localising to pain, there are a few more significant responses that patients may exhibit. These are described in the section of this chapter focusing on the Glasgow Coma Scale. In the AVPU system a response to pain is recorded as present if any response to a painful stimuli is exhibited by the patient, and as absent if no response is exhibited; where no response is exhibited then the person is described as being unresponsive or scoring U on the AVPU scale.

Methods of applying a painful stimulus

Painful stimuli can be classified as either peripheral or central. Peripheral stimulation is that which is applied to the extremities such as the hands, whereas central stimulation is that which is applied to core structures of the body. Both peripheral and central stimulation have a role to play in assessing the person's level of consciousness. Light peripheral stimulation such as touching a person's arm can be used initially to assess if a person is arousable before attempting more painful central stimulation, which is used to formally assess a person's response to painful stimuli using the Glasgow Coma Scale. Several methods have been described for the application of central painful stimuli. These include:

- Squeezing the trapezium muscle at the point where the shoulder meets the neck. This is currently probably the most accepted method for applying central painful stimuli. Manipulation of the neck, however, is contraindicated if there is any history of neck trauma. The presence of any medical devices in the neck, such as vascular access devices or tracheotomy tubes, require the operator to exercise extreme caution and clinical judgement about the appropriateness of this technique.
- Applying pressure over the supraorbital notch. Here the thumb is used to palpate the supraorbital margin. A notch is felt close to the nose in most subjects. Once located, pressure is then applied to this notch to elicit a painful response. However, this method should not be used if there is a possibility of facial fractures or fragile bones.
- Sternal friction rub, which involves rubbing the knuckles of the examiner's clenched fist along the sternum of the patient. This is a particularly painful technique and therefore less suitable for repeated testing. In many centres this technique has lost popularity.

Whenever a response to pain is sought practitioners must use only the minimal amount of force needed to precipitate a response, in concert with sound clinical judgement.

The AVPU scale

While the AVPU score is useful in quickly classifying a patient's level of consciousness, it is also important not to forget that this is a relatively crude tool and changes in a person's level of consciousness can be quite subtle. There is a significant difference between a person who is holding a coherent conversation and a person who is alert but seriously confused. Patients who present with new–onset confusion or are combative are also likely to be acutely ill and this finding should never be ignored until a cause has been identified and treatment provided if necessary. Patients who have developed an altered level of consciousness will need to have their neurological function monitored more closely, which can be done using the Glasgow Coma Scale.

Glasgow Coma Scale

The Glasgow Coma Scale is a tool that was devised by Teasdale and Jennett in 1974. Their aim was to provide a simple-to-use tool that was able to accurately quantify a person's level of consciousness and provide a framework through which changes in consciousness could be tracked. The scale uses key markers of consciousness to quantify the patient's condition. The score that is derived from the scale is made up of three components: eye opening (4 potential points), verbal response (5 potential points) and motor response (6 potential points), with the total score achievable being 15 (Box 3.4). As different versions of the scale have been introduced over time it is important to express the scale as being out of 15, so the score should be recorded as, for example, 13/15. Whenever the score is less than 15, as is the example, the separate components of the score should be recorded along with the total, that is, GCS E3 V4 M6 total 13/15.

You will note that the lowest score achievable is 3. It is therefore possible for a patient with score of 3 to be either deeply unconscious or dead. A score of 8 or less is often seen as an indication to intubate the patient, whereas a score of 12 indicates a significant pathology.

BOX 3.4 The Glasgow Coma Scale for adults

The Glasgow Coma Scale is scored between 3 and 15, 3 being the worst, and 15 the best. It comprises three parameters: best eye response, best verbal response, best motor response. The definition of these parameters is given below.

Best eye response (4)

4 Eyes open spontaneously
3 Eyes opening to verbal command
2 Eyes opening to pain
1 No eye opening

Best verbal response (5)

5 Orientated
4 Confused
3 Inappropriate words
2 Incomprehensible sounds
1 No verbal response

(Continued)

(Continued)

Best motor response (6)

6 Obeys commands
5 Localising pain
4 Normal flexion to pain
3 Abnormal flexion to pain
2 Extension to pain
1 No motor response

The Glasgow Coma Scale is used worldwide and is well respected, although some have reported that there can be discrepancies between scores made by different healthcare professionals who rate the same patient at the same time, raising questions about its interreliability (Gill et al., 2004). Others have found a good degree of interreliability (Juarez and Lyons 1996; Cohen, 2009). The reasons for these discrepancies are likely to be various. One important consideration is health professionals' understanding of the terms used in the Glasgow Coma Scale. While many of the terms used in the scale are obvious, others require clarification or have specific meanings, and to combat the problem of interreliability it is necessary to ensure that there is clarity of understanding for each of the terms that are included in the scale. To assist with this, definitions of the key terms are provided in Table 3.2.

TABLE 3.2   *Meaning of the terms used in the Glasgow Coma Scale*

Term	Meaning	Score
Eye responses		
Eyes open *spontaneously*	Means without any stimulation	4
Eyes opening to *verbal command*	Means when spoken to, e.g. 'Hello can you hear me, can you open your eyes?'	3
Eyes opening to *pain*	Means eyes open to painful stimulus. Assess light rousing stimulus first, then central stimulation, e.g. trapezium squeeze, supra-orbital pressure or sternal friction rub	2
No eye opening	Eyes do not open at all	1
Verbal responses		
Orientated	Means the person knows who they are (name), who you are (nurse, doctor, etc.), where they are (hospital), time frame (day, year)	5
Confused	Means able to carry out a conversation but not fully oriented as above	4

TABLE 3.2 *(Continued)*

Term	Meaning	Score
Inappropriate words	Means that recognised words are uttered but not in the form of an exchange. This does not mean swear words	3
Incomprehensible sounds	Means grunts, groans or incomprehensible words	2
No verbal response	Means no vocalisation, even in response to pain	1
Motor responses		
Obeys commands	The patient is able to do as you ask, e.g. 'Place both arms out in front of you with your palms upwards and close your eyes.' This also allows you to test strength in the arms	6
Localising pain	Means that attempts are made to remove the painful stimulus. Arms are brought up and cross the midline of the body in an attempt to remove a central painful stimulus	5
Normal flexion to pain	Flexes (bends) arm at the elbow without rotation of the wrist, in response to a central painful stimulus	4
Abnormal flexion to pain	Flexes (bends) arm at the elbow *with* rotation of the wrist (Figure 3.1a) (decorticate posturing) in response to a central painful stimulus	3
Extension to pain	Extends (straightens) arms with inward rotation of the arm (decerebrate posturing) (Figure 3.1b), in response to a central painful stimulus	2
No motor response	No motor response seen even in response to a painful stimulus	1

Caveats to using the Glasgow Coma Scale

- It is important to remember that you should score the best response that is seen.
- Responses to painful stimuli should be completed simultaneously; do not repeat the application of pain separately for each of the eyes, voice and motor domains.
- If the person's eyes are closed as a result of trauma, swelling, surgery, etc., then record the eyes as closed. In some centres this is abbreviated as a 'C' on the neurological observations chart.
- Intubated patients will not be able to speak; record 'T' for tube on the neurological observations chart.
- Patients with previously documented dysphasia will also not be able to speak; document 'D' on the neurological observations chart.

In addition to the Glasgow Coma Scale, the ability of the patient to move their limbs with normal strength, to have normal sensation in the body and normal pupil responses is also a part of the deeper neurological assessment.

(A) Decorticate posturing

(B) Deceberate posturing

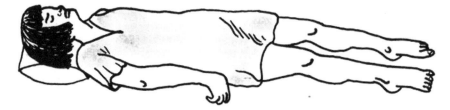

FIGURE 3.1   *Responses to painful stimulus.*

Capillary refill

Capillary refill, time is a test of how quickly the capillary beds refill after blood has been evacuated from them. It is a measure of vasoconstriction and can be an early sign that the circulation to the periphery of the body is reduced, with blood being directed towards more central vital organs. To test the capillary refill time:

1   Elevate a person's hand above the level of the heart.
2   Note the colour of the nail bed.
3   Squeeze the nail bed quite firmly between your thumb and forefinger for five seconds.
4   Then release the pressure and time how long it takes for the colour to return to its previous state. It may be helpful to compare against another finger.

A normal capillary refill is two seconds or less. Refill that takes longer than two seconds is abnormal and indicates shunting of blood away from the periphery. Occasionally however, capillary refill will be abnormally brisk. This can indicate vasodilatation and may be a feature of sepsis or carbon dioxide retention. Capillary refill will normally be reduced where a patient has been exposed to cold temperatures and this must be taken into consideration. If the fingers are unavailable for the assessment of capillary refill, alternative sites such as the tip of the nose or the sternum can be utilised.

Pulse

While initially describing how to check a pulse may seem obvious, a considerable amount of information that can be gained from a correct pulse check is often lost or its significance not understood by the assessor. A pulse can be checked at many sites in the body, and those most relevant in the care of acutely ill are the radial pulse in the wrists and the carotid pulse in the neck. The main difference between these two pulses is that the radial pulse is considered to be a peripheral pulse while the carotid is classed as a central pulse. This distinction is important, as at times of low blood pressure the radial pulse may become unreliable. Blood is directed away from the periphery of the body and thus the radial pulse may become undetectable when the blood pressure is critically low, despite the heart continuing to beat. It is for this reason that only central pulses should be assessed to determine the presence or absence of a pulse when a person is experiencing an acute life-threatening event. Even then caution needs to be exercised when assessing the carotid pulse as this can be difficult for the inexperienced practitioner, particularly when the stress of an emergency situation complicates the assessment.

When assessing a patient's pulse you should be interested in:

- Pulse rate
- Rhythm of the pulse
- Volume of the pulse.

The pulse rate is the number of times in a minute that a pressure wave of blood can be felt. In health, the pulse rate should correlate with the heart rate. However, if an arrhythmia develops or there are a number of ectopic beats the heart rate may be different from the pulse rate as the heart may contract when empty, producing a heart beat but no effective cardiac output for that beat. When this occurs it is called a pulse deficit. A normal pulse rate is between 60 and 100 beats per minute, with pulses of less than 60 beats per minute described as a bradycardia, and rates greater than 100 beats per minute described as a tachycardia. The patient's pulse rate, though, needs to be interpreted in the light of the circumstances of the patient. A young athletic individual may have a slow resting heart rate (<60 beats per minute) though this is of little clinical significance. Likewise a person who has just undertaken vigorous exercise is likely to have a fast heart rate (>100 beats per minute) though again this is of little clinical significance. Heart rates of less than 40 beats per minute are always concerning and warrant immediate assessment by a physician.

The rhythm of the pulse relates to how regular or irregular the pulse feels. While in health the pulse should be regular, some young, healthy individuals experience a cyclical increase and decrease in heart rate, which is normally associated with the pattern of breathing. This is a phenomenon known as sinus arrhythmia and is a benign finding in the young, healthy individual. Other causes of an irregular pulse are more sinister arrhythmias. Any patient with an irregular pulse should have an electrocardiogram (ECG) in order to classify the arrhythmia (see Chapter 6). Some of the most common causes of an irregular pulse are atrial fibrillation, premature contractions and second-degree heart block. It is worth noting if the irregularity in pulse rate is constantly present or occurs intermittently.

The volume of the pulse refers to how strong or weak the pulse feels. Essentially, the volume of the pulse is governed by the difference between the systolic and diastolic blood pressure. A weak-volume pulse can indicate peripheral vasoconstriction, low stroke volume, heart failure or hypovolaemia. A full-volume pulse is caused by an increase in stroke volume or a reduction in peripheral vascular resistance, for example in those who are vasodilated. Full-volume pulses are often seen in patients who have fever, carbon dioxide retention, neurological insult or sepsis. Occasionally, the volume of the pulse will vary from beat to beat. You are most likely to feel this in patients with atrial fibrillation, although it can also occur in patients with heart failure. The correct term to describe this variation is pulsus alternans.

Respiratory assessment

The respiratory system is very sensitive to the changes that occur during an episode of acute illness and as such is a good marker of underlying pathology. When assessing respiratory function, there are five things that you should consider:

- Respiratory rate
- Rhythm or pattern of respiration
- Depth of breaths
- Symmetry of chest expansion
- Amount of effort invested in breathing.

The respiratory rate is the number of breaths a patient takes per minute. A normal respiratory rate is between 12 and 20 breaths per minute. Respiratory rates over 20 breaths per minute are referred to as tachypnoea and rates of less than 12 breaths per minute are classed as bradypnoea. Patients have a degree of voluntary control over their respiratory rate and thus, it is important that you assess a patient's respiratory rate without telling them that you are about to do so. This will prevent any conscious or subconscious change in the respiratory rate or pattern. For this reason, it is best to assess the patient's respiratory rate while feeling the pulse so the patient believes that you are taking their pulse and does not change their respiratory picture. Count the number of breaths that the patient takes over a one-minute period. One breath is classed as one cycle of inspiration and expiration.

While you are counting the respiratory rate, note also the pattern of respiration. This should be regular. Irregular breathing is abnormal and may indicate a serious underlying problem. The amount of air that moves with each breath is referred to as the depth of breathing. At times of exercise both respiratory rate and depth increases to compensate for the additional oxygen used by muscles. There are a number of characteristic changes that can occur, both in respiratory pattern and depth, and these are summarised in Figure 3.2.

Look to see if both sides of the chest are moving symmetrically with each breath. Asymmetrical chest movement can be a sign of serious lung pathology. Patients who have received pneumonectomy will obviously have asymmetrical chest movement. The amount of effort or work that the person has to put into breathing should also be considered. Normal breathing is effortless. If a person is having to sit up or forward to breathe comfortably then this is abnormal. The majority of the work of breathing is undertaken by the diaphragm, hence normal breathing is referred to as diaphragmatic. The intercostal muscles also contribute to the mechanism of breathing; this is normally reserved to increase ventilation during times of illness or exercise. A patient who is resting and using intercostal muscles probably has some form of respiratory problem. The patient who is using accessory muscles of respiration, such as the sternocleidomastoids, definitely has a respiratory problem.

Oxygen saturation

Oxygen saturation is a test which measures the amount of oxygen bound to the haemoglobin in the red blood cells. The main benefit of oxygen saturation assessment is that it is non-invasive and can detect hypoxaemia

Pattern of breathing	Name and clinical significance
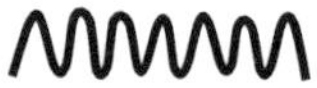 MMMM	*Eupnoea:* Normal regular breathing at a rate of 12–20 breaths per minute
⅃_⅃	*Apnoea:* Pauses in breathing lasting 15 seconds or longer. Seen in opioid overdoses, sleep apnoea and respiratory arrest
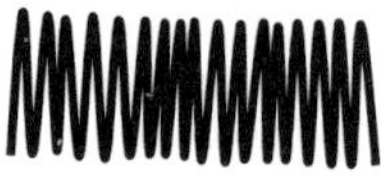 MMMMMMMM	*Kussmaul's:* Rapid deep breathing, occurs in metabolic acidosis as carbon dioxide is blown off to restore the pH of the blood. Diabetic ketoacidosis is a common cause
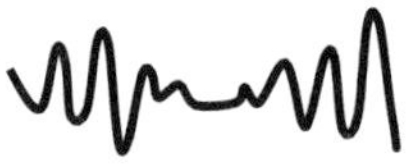 ⅗⅂⅌⅃	*Cheyne–Stokes:* Crescendo–decrescendo breathing often associated with end-stage disease. Occurs in metabolic disarrangement and central nervous system (CNS) insults
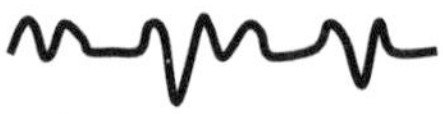 ⅍⅌⅟	*Ataxic:* Irregular pattern of breathing, depth of breaths may be irregular also. Can degenerate into agonal gasps. CNS insult is a common cause
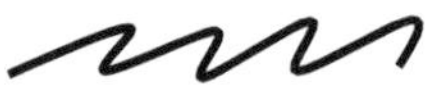 ⅃⅃⅃	*Apneustic:* Increased inspiratory time with short expiratory time. May sound like grunting. Caused by a CNS insult
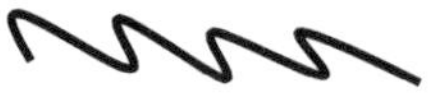 ⅏⅏⅏	*Pronged expiratory phase:* Occurs in obstructive airway diseases, such as chronic obstructive pulmonary disease, and acutely in asthma

FIGURE 3.2   *Patterns of breathing.*

earlier than most clinicians. Until the advent of pulse oximetry, the only way to establish the amount of oxygen contained within the blood was through arterial blood gas (ABG) analysis and, to this day, ABG remains the gold standard assessment.

Pulse oximetry measures the amount of oxygen attached to haemoglobin by shining both red and infrared light through the tissues. A light sensor detects the amount of red light that is transmitted through the tissues. The pulse oximeter is able to detect when a pulse of blood is passed over the sensor and this allows it to differentiate between arterial and venous blood in most circumstances. As oxygenated blood is more bright red in colour than deoxygenated blood, the pulse oximeter is essentially measuring the colour of the blood and using this to calculate the percentage of haemoglobin which is saturated with oxygen. Normal values are 94–100% with levels of 93% or less indicating hypoxia. When levels fall below 90% the patient is very unwell and when levels fall below 85% the situation is an emergency. Some patients, notably those with chronic obstructive pulmonary disease (COPD), will have become accustomed to lower levels of oxygen in their blood and readings that would cause tremendous concern in the general population will be the COPD patient's norm. This said, however, any low oxygen saturation level requires careful assessment, with the additional assessment of ABG in this group of patients. Low oxygen saturation can only be considered to be chronic when it has previously been shown to be low. Any sudden change in a person's oxygen saturation of 3% or more is always concerning and warrants a full review of the patient no matter what their diagnosis.

One of the limitations of pulse oximetry is that it provides information only about the saturation of oxygen in a patient's blood, but it does not determine how much carbon dioxide is dissolved in the blood. For this reason, pulse oximetry may need to be combined with ABG assessment if a full picture of the patient's respiratory function is to be established. The accuracy of pulse oximetry is influenced by a number of factors, which are logically understood if the mechanism pulse oximetry is understood (see Box 3.5).

BOX 3.5 Factors that cause artefacts in pulse oximetry tests

- Problems with blood supply to the location of the sensor – this may be arterial or venous obstruction:

  - Low blood pressure
  - Injury proximal to the site of the sensor
  - Pre-existing arterial or venous disease
  - Cardiac arrhythmia

- Problems with the concentration of haemoglobin in the blood:

  - Anaemia (low haemoglobin, false high result)
  - Polycythaemia (too much haemoglobin, false low result)

- Dysfunctional haemoglobin:

  - Carboxyhaemoglobin (carbon monoxide bound to haemoglobin in place of oxygen, false high result)
  - Methaemoglobinaemia (poor ability of the haemoglobin to give out oxygen)

- Problems with light passage/absorption:

  - Dirty skin, dried blood, oil or dark nail polish
  - Bright external lights

It is essential to interpret the pulse oximeter in the light of any oxygen therapy that the patient is receiving – a reading of 92% while a patient is breathing room air is less worrying than a patient with a result of 92% while breathing 100% oxygen. Pulse oximeters are not well calibrated at low levels (<85%) and so may provide an inaccurate result. Small drops in oxygen saturation at lower levels (<85%) hold the same significance as larger drops at the higher end of the scale as they indicate significant escalating hypoxia. Refer to the manufacturer's instructions for information on calibration and the specific methods that you should use to record a patient's oxygen saturation in your practice setting.

Blood pressure

The recording of a blood pressure, like taking a pulse, is something that most clinicians are familiar with. Yet the advent of automated blood pressure devices has resulted in many professionals becoming deskilled in the accurate manual recording of blood pressure. As with checking a pulse manually, there is a lot more information that can be gained by taking a blood pressure manually than can be obtained from an automated blood pressure machine. At the same time it is important to widen one's view of blood pressure to include more than the systolic pressure over the diastolic pressure, as the mean arterial pressure and the pulse pressure are also important considerations when caring for the acutely ill.

In order for blood to circulate effectively, it must be under pressure. Blood pressure is created by the perfusion triad. This is described in full in Chapter 5 but essentially consists of blood volume, vascular resistance and cardiac output. Blood pressure is the pressure that blood exerts on the inner arterial walls. There are two blood pressures that can be measured – the systolic and diastolic pressures. The systolic pressure represents the peak pressure that is experienced by a blood vessel and coincides with the heartbeat, hence it is termed systolic. The diastolic blood pressure is the resting pressure and represents the least pressure exerted on the blood vessel and coincides with the resting stages in the cardiac cycle, hence termed diastolic.

It is difficult to state what a normal blood pressure is in acute care, as it is a change in blood pressure that is probably more important than the actual numbers that are seen. Traditionally, the systolic blood pressure was seen as the all important number and to some degree this remains true today. In terms of interpreting the systolic pressure an arbitrary number of 90 mmHg has been set by many as an indicator of failing blood pressure. The 90 mmHg threshold, though, assumes that the person had a healthy blood pressure prior to becoming unwell. 'Take, for example, a healthy person with a systolic pressure of 120 mmHg. If they lost blood volume and subsequently their blood pressure fell to 90 mmHg then there is a 30 mmHg drop in their blood pressure. Now consider a patient who was previously hypertensive with a blood pressure of 180 mmHg who experienced a drop in their blood pressure to a systolic of 90 mmHg. Their blood pressure will have dropped by a staggering 90 mmHg. This dramatic fall in blood pressure is likely to result in a serious haemodynamic challenge to the body as it is equivalent to the healthy person dropping their systolic blood pressure from 120 mmHg to 30 mmHg. For this reason, in patients who were previously hypertensive, a drop of only 30 mmHg in the systolic blood pressure is significant.

When estimating blood pressure, it is important that you are using equipment that has been validated for clinical use by the British Hypertension Society (2004) and that it has been properly calibrated. Guidelines on the estimation of blood pressure have been published by the European Hypertension Society (O' Brien et al., 2003) and every person who records blood pressure should be familiar with them. To gain the most accurate picture of a patient's blood pressure the patient should have been sitting resting in that position for at least five minutes. The European Hypertension Society guidelines are, however, directed at an optimal technique for the detection of hypertension. During an episode of acute illness the blood pressure is being measured as a marker of illness severity. In this circumstance it may be irrelevant to require the patient to sit for five minutes prior to recording a blood pressure. The first time that a blood pressure is taken from a patient, it should be taken in both arms to help rule out vascular pathology such as aortic coarctation (a narrowing of the aorta). The blood pressure can vary in both arms, but a difference of 20 mmHg systolic or 10 mmHg diastolic is clinically significant and warrants investigation if it is reproducible.

The blood pressure cuff should be placed on the patient's arm that is free from restrictive clothing. It is important to use a cuff of the correct size. The inflatable bladder of a blood pressure cuff should cover 80–100% of the circumference of the arm. Bladders that are too small, with <80% coverage, result in an overestimation of the blood pressure and cuffs that are too large, with >100% coverage, result in an underestimation of the blood pressure. The bladder should be positioned so that the brachial artery is at its centre. The patient's arm should be supported at the level of the heart, as an elevated or dependent limb can affect the result.

The brachial pulse should then be palpated and the cuff inflated until the pulse can no longer be felt; this is the estimated systolic pressure. It is important to perform this step as the presence of an auscultatory gap can result in significant underestimation of the systolic blood pressure if this assessment is not performed. The cuff should then be deflated and the stethoscope positioned over the brachial artery. The stethoscope should not be placed under the cuff. The cuff should then be inflated to 30 mmHg above the estimated systolic pressure. The air should then be released from the cuff slowly at about 2 mmHg per second. While the pressure in the cuff is above that of the blood, no pulse is palpable and no sounds can be heard at the brachial artery. While normal, unrestricted blood flow is silent the application of an inflated blood pressure cuff creates turbulence in the blood flow and this is audible with a stethoscope. As the air is allowed to escape from the cuff the pressure in the cuff gradually decreases. When the blood pressure equalises with the pressure in the cuff, blood is able to pass the inflated cuff in time with cardiac systole but not at diastole. A sound is heard each time a pulse of blood passes the cuff. These sounds, of which there are five phases, are referred to as the Korotkoff sounds, named after Russian physician Nikolai Korotkoff who first described them. After the initial sound is heard (phase 2) the sounds should then become louder (phase 3) and then muffle (phase 4) till the point where they eventually disappear (phase 5). The point of disappearance indicates the point at which blood flow is no longer turbulent and thus cannot be heard. The descriptor phase 1 is used to describe the silence created by an absence of blood flow when the cuff pressure is greater than the systolic blood pressure.

When a continuous tapping sound can be heard (phase 2 sounds) this is the point of the systolic pressure. Record the point at which this is heard to the nearest 2 mmHg on the scale. Then continue to listen to the Korotkoff sounds. When the sounds disappear (phase 5), note this on the scale to the nearest 2 mmHg as this represents the diastolic pressure. In some patients, sounds can be heard all the way down to the point where the cuff is emptied. In these patients the point of muffling (phase 4) will need to be used to represent the diastolic pressure. This should be recorded to the nearest 2 mmHg along with the fact that phase 4 was used. Always record what the blood pressure was to the nearest 2 mmHg, never round the blood pressure to the nearest 5 or 10 mmHg.

Once the systolic and diastolic blood pressures are known, it is possible to calculate the mean arterial pressure and the pulse pressure. The mean arterial pressure is the estimated perfusion pressure at the level of the organs. For organs to be perfused correctly this should not fall below 70 mmHg. The mean arterial pressure is calculated using the following formula:

$$\frac{\text{Systolic} + (\text{Diastolic} \times 2)}{3}$$

Pulse pressure is the difference between the systolic pressure and the diastolic pressure. To calculate the pulse pressure, simply subtract the diastolic pressure from the systolic pressure. The normal pulse pressure is 30–40 mmHg and any widening or narrowing of the pulse pressure can indicate signs of acute illness. The pulse pressure is created by the amount of systemic vascular resistance and the stroke volume (the amount of blood ejected from the left ventricle in one beat). As a general rule, factors which affect the stroke volume affect the systolic pressure, while changes in vascular resistance affect the diastolic pressure (Adam and Osborne, 2005).

When vasoconstriction occurs, as is the case in the compensation for a reduced blood volume, the diastolic pressure will rise slightly in the early stages of shock, illustrating activation of vasoconstriction. As an increasing volume of fluid is lost the cardiac output will also become reduced. The net effect of these combined problems is a narrowed pulse pressure (Figure 3.3). Likewise, if the stroke volume is reduced due to, say, arrhythmia then the pulse pressure will narrow. In patients in a vasodilated state with increased cardiac output, such as sepsis and carbon dioxide retention, the pulse pressure can widen significantly (Figure 3.3C).

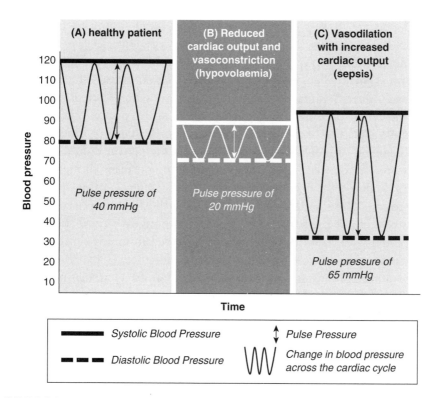

FIGURE 3.3   *Examples of changes seen in pulse pressure.*

Assessment of pulse pressure is a complicated endeavour as it is dependent on a number of interrelated factors. You will need to be mindful of this and recognise that pulse pressure needs to be interpreted as part of a wider PSA. The most important factors to recognise are that both a wide and narrow pulse pressure are abnormal as are significant changes in pulse pressure.

Pulsus paradoxus is a phenomenon when the blood pressure changes with inspiration and expiration. While a degree of pulsus paradoxus (<10 mmHg) is seen in healthy individuals, any increase above 10 mmHg is pathological and indicates some form of intra-thoracic pathology. In pulsus paradoxus the drop in systolic blood pressure normally occurs in time with inspiration. This factor cannot be detected with a non-invasive, automated blood pressure machine and requires either manual estimation of blood pressure using a sphygmomanometer or an invasive blood pressure monitor. Pathological pulsus paradoxus occurs when there is a restriction to blood flow, due to a pressure change within the chest. This may be due to pericardial tamponade, tension pneumothorax or hyperinflation of the chest during an acute asthma attack. Reverse pulsus paradoxus can occur in ventilated patients and this has the potential to reduce cardiac output.

A final point of note is to consider the effects of patient position on blood pressure. It is possible for the patient lying supine to maintain a healthy blood pressure despite a significantly reduced effective circulating volume. It is simpler for the body to maintain blood pressure in the supine position as the challenges that are placed on blood pressure by gravity are largely eliminated. It may be useful in some cases where there is doubt over the true blood pressure to make the patient sit up and check the blood pressure again. This will help to reveal an orthostatic (positional) drop, which can indicate volume depletion. Ideally, the person should have their blood pressure checked in the lying or standing position, though standing an acutely ill patient may be impractical and making them sit up is a good compromise. The standard definition of an orthostatic drop is a reduction in systolic blood pressure by 20 mmHg, although this will need to be interpreted with caution if the patient is moved from a lying to a sitting, not standing, position. Orthostatic hypotension occurs in hypovolaemia and in other conditions that lead to reduced effective circulating volume. Orthostatic hypotension may also feature as a result of damage to the sympathetic nervous system, for example through the presence of autonomic neuropathy in patients with diabetes. It may occur in patients who are taking antihypertensive medicines. In pregnant patients, the blood pressure can drop significantly if the gravid uterus is allowed to compress the inferior vena cava. To avoid this, pregnant patients will always need to have their blood pressure measured while sitting or lying reclined to the left.

Fluid balance

Dehydration is a common problem among hospitalised patients. The accurate monitoring of a patient's fluid balance is necessary to prevent this. To do this you must first calculate the person's basic fluid requirement for 24 hours (Chapter 5). The fluid intake must then be assessed against this and supported if intake falls below this level. Fluid intake should be balanced against fluid loss from urine, vomiting, wound exudates or drains. It is normal for the healthy body to lose 500 mL of fluid a day in what is termed insensible loss, that is, fluid lost in faeces, sweat and breathing. At time of illness this may be increased and will need to be compensated for. At the end of each 24-hour period, the fluid balance should be calculated and a plan to correct any problems put in place. Laboratory assessment of urea and electrolytes will supplement this decision making.

Urine output

Urine output is a sensitive marker of organ perfusion and fluid status. At times of haemodynamic compromise renal perfusion is reduced and water reabsorption in the kidneys is increased. Both these actions cause a reduction in the amount of urine produced. Clinically this is seen as a reduction in the urine output. The body must continuously produce urine in order to rid itself of non-volatile acids. Failure to produce adequate volumes of urine can result in metabolic acidosis. The normal urine output should be in excess of 0.5 mL/per kg of weight per hour. Anything less than this is classed as oliguria and can lead to acute kidney injury.

There are a number of causes of oliguria in addition to haemodynamic compromise. When a patient presents with apparent oliguria you should first try to establish if this is true oliguria. Rule out the possibility of urinary retention, which can be detected through the use of bladder palpation, percussion or bladder scanning. In patients with a catheter in situ check to see that the catheter is not being bypassed or has become blocked. Where a reduction in urine output is identified or predicted, drugs which are nephrotoxic should be stopped. These include all non-steroidal anti-inflammatory drugs, angiotensin-converting enzyme inhibitors and some antibiotics. At this stage, note that oliguria in the presence of haemodynamic compromise should be treated initially with fluid replacement and never diuretics as these are likely to worsen the overall situation. However, when the reduced urine output is caused by a problem with the heart caution must be exercised when administrating additional fluid as there is a real risk of precipitating or worsening heart failure. In this situation it is usual to halve the dose of fluid given if the person is considered to be volume depleted, while addressing the cardiac problem that has presented.

In a clinical setting assessing a patient's urine output can be challenging, particularly if the patient is not catheterised. It may therefore be easier to calculate the four-hourly urine output and assess this. Educating patients in the need for monitoring their urine output will also help in ensuring compliance. A patient's minimum urine output should be calculated and displayed on their assessment chart. For patients where there is concern over their urine output, a catheter should be passed so that the urine output can be monitored more closely; ideally this catheter should be connected to a catheter bag with an hourly measurement device. For patients who are not catheterised, weighing their urine on a tared scale to account for the weight of the bottle or bed pan is a good alternative. One millilitre of urine is equivalent to 1g.

The opposite of oliguria is polyuria, which is defined as the production of greater than 3L of urine in 24 hours. By far the most common cause of polyuria is hyperglycaemia in the poorly controlled diabetic patient, though there are other causes such as diabetes insipidus and high-output renal failure. It is important to identify patients with polyuria as they can quickly become dehydrated and experience haemodynamic compromise as a result of hypovolaemia.

Vomiting and other outputs

Do not forget to ask whether a patient has vomited and check any sites from which fluid may be lost such as wound dressings or drains. Both these points are important for a number of reasons. Firstly, any fluid loss from the body needs to be recorded so that it can be taken into account when calculating the patient's fluid requirements. Secondly, patients who vomit lose chloride ions, and excessive vomiting can result in not only dehydration but also metabolic alkalosis which may require correction. Thirdly, vomiting is a sign of illness in itself and its presence warrants investigation. Vomiting will also make the patient feel ill and you may consider the use of antiemetic agents to improve the patient's experience and reduce the risk of further fluid loss.

Temperature

Body temperature can vary for a variety of reasons. While many healthcare professionals associate infection with a raised temperature, there are many other causes of this, including other inflammatory conditions, tissue injury, malignancy, hyperthyroidism and drugs. As well as becoming elevated, body temperature can fall below the normal range. The most common cause of this is environmental exposure to cold, although heat can be lost from the body after surgery or as a result of evaporation of wound exudates, which can be a particular problem in people with serious burn injuries. Hypothyroidism is an additional cause of a low temperature. Deviation from normal body temperature places a number of challenges on the body. High temperatures increase both oxygen demand and fluid requirements. Low temperatures suppress normal body functions.

The normal body temperature varies over a 24-hour period, being at its lowest in the early hours of the morning and highest in the early evening. During this time it is possible to observe a normal variance of 1°C. The exact temperature range for the healthy human is the subject of disagreement in the literature. A range of 36.3–37.1°C seems an acceptable range to work with. When temperature rises to 40°C or above the person is said to be hyperthermic and when temperature falls below 35°C hypothermia is said to have occurred. There is a range of devices that can be used to measure a patient's temperature. The once popular glass thermometer has now largely been replaced by chemical strips or electronic devices. You should always read the manufacturer's instructions for any device that you are expected to use.

While less precise, the temperature of a patient's extremities gives an indication of how well the body as a whole is being perfused. Cold extremities indicate vasoconstriction, whereas warm extremities indicate vasodilatation. It is important to rule out peripheral vascular disease before using this sign, or else spurious results may be obtained. Likewise patients who have recently been in the cold are likely to have cold extremities. To assess the extremity temperature, touch the patient on each leg with the back of your hand to assess its temperature.

Pain

Pain is a natural part of many illness states. It is a warning to us from our body that something is not right. The cause of pain should be identified and appropriate analgesia administered with its effects monitored. Specific pain charts exist to track a patient's experience of pain and full use of such tools is advocated to manage a patient's pain optimally. A simple way of quantifying a patient's pain is to ask where their pain sits on a continuous scale of 0–10, with 0 meaning no pain at all and 10 being the worst pain imaginable (Holdgate et al., 2003). This can then be documented and a patient's response to analgesia monitored. It may also be useful to show a patient a list of words that may be used to describe the type of pain that the patient has (see Box 3.6).

BOX 3.6 Words used to describe pain

Tender	Dull
Crushing	Sore
Squeezing	Aching
Stabbing	Gnawing
Sharp	Ripping
Burning	Feels like a weight
Like an electric shock	Pressure
Throbbing	A discomfort
Cramping	

Conclusion

Being able to successfully identify those who are acutely ill is an essential skill for those involved in caring for patients. All too often patient deterioration is missed as a full PSA was not made. Reliance on isolated values of vital signs which appear to be within the arbitrarily set normal ranges will not assist in identifying the majority of those who are acutely ill.

Improving practice involves adopting a structured and standardised PSA approach that is grounded in a physiological understanding of the changes that occur during an episode of acute illness. Decision-support tools such as EWS systems are useful adjuncts, but they do have limitations and users of such tools should be aware of what these are.

Finally, any assessment is only as good as the quality of the information that it is based upon. Using correct techniques to collect data is essential if decisions appropriate to the patient's needs are to be made.

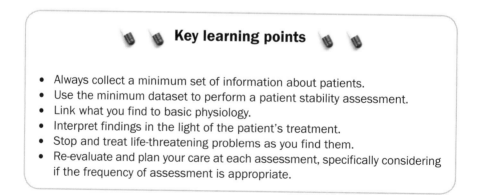

Key learning points

- Always collect a minimum set of information about patients.
- Use the minimum dataset to perform a patient stability assessment.
- Link what you find to basic physiology.
- Interpret findings in the light of the patient's treatment.
- Stop and treat life-threatening problems as you find them.
- Re-evaluate and plan your care at each assessment, specifically considering if the frequency of assessment is appropriate.

🔋 🔋 Self-assessment questions 🔋 🔋

1   Which one of the following observations is not part of the minimum data-set that should be obtained as a part of screening acutely ill patients?

   A   Urine output
   B   Respiratory rate
   C   Blood pressure
   D   Peak expiratory flow rate
   C   Pulse rate

2   A patient for whom you are caring has observations of respiratory rate 18 breaths per minute; pulse 82 beats per minute; BP 112/65 mmHg. Which one of the following statements is true?

   A   The patient has observations which suggest that they are haemodynamically stable
   B   There is insufficient information provided in order to make a reasoned assessment of this patient's needs
   C   The patient is likely to be physiologically unstable
   D   A doctor or outreach team should be made aware of this patient
   E   The patient should receive four-hourly observations

3   Screening tests in the acutely ill:

   A   Can be completed and interpreted in isolation from other screening tests
   B   Consist of respiratory rate, pulse and blood pressure only
   C   Will always be abnormal in the acutely ill
   D   Provide an early indication of the presence of acute illness when used correctly
   E   Provide a definitive picture of what is going on in a patient

4   Patients who have a normal early warning score will:

   A   Always be stable
   B   Likely to be stable, but vigilance is still required as signs of compensation can be masked
   C   Need ongoing screening assessments every four hours
   D   Need ongoing screening assessments every hour
   E   Need no further assessment in a 24-hour period

5   You discover that a patient has a respiratory rate of 23 breaths per minute and an SaO_2 of 90%. Which one of the following is the correct course of action to take?

   A   Stop the screening tests and give oxygen
   B   Carry on with the screening until all tests are completed
   C   Stop the screening tests and immediately summon help

(Continued)

(Continued)

    D   Calculate the early warning score based on these clearly abnormal values

    E   Pause the screening to give oxygen, complete the screening and summon help simultaneously if possible.

6   Mean arterial pressure represents:

    A   The difference between the systolic and diastolic pressure
    B   The pulse pressure
    C   The perfusion pressure of blood at the tissue level
    D   Both B and C
    E   The osmotic pressure in the venous system

7   Which one of the following drugs that may be prescribed can inhibit a patient's ability to compensate for an episode of acute illness?

    A   Paracetamol
    B   Sodium chloride 0.9%
    C   Lisinopril
    D   Salbutamol
    C   Aminophylline

8   A widened pulse pressure is a sign of:

    A   Vasodilation
    B   Vasoconstriction
    C   Hypotension
    D   Hypertension
    C   Hypercapnia

Answers

1D, 2B, 3D, 4B, 5E, 6C, 7C, 8A.

Further reading

Epstein, O., Perkin, D., Cookson, J. and de Bono, D. (2003) *Clinical Examination*, 3rd edn. Edinburgh: Mosby.
This is a text that provides more depth on how to clinically examine patients and make sense of the findings.

O'Brien, E., Asmar, R., Beilin, L., Imai, Y., Mallion, J., Mancia, G., Mengden, T., Myers, M., Padfield, P., Palatini, P., Parati, G., Pickering, T., Redon, J., Staessen, J., Stergiou, G. and Verdecchia, P. on behalf of the European Society of Hypertension Working Group on Blood Pressure Monitoring (2003) 'European Society of Hypertension recommendations for conventional, ambulatory and home blood pressure measurement', *Journal of Hypertension*, 21: 821–48.
This is an important guideline that describes how blood pressure should be measured. As such it is an essential read for any person involved in measuring blood pressure.

4

Problems with the airway and breathing

Chapter aims

By the end of this chapter you should be able to:

- Describe the anatomy of the respiratory system
- Recognise problems with the airway and breathing
- Take action to secure the airway
- Assist senior clinicians with advanced airway procedures
- Understand the development of breathing problems
- Take action to support breathing

Breathing is fundamentally important to life and without the ability to breathe the body will soon die. As a minimum for effective breathing a person must have a clear airway and functioning lungs. Other factors will also impact on the effectiveness of the airway and breathing, such as neurological status and homeostatic stability. At times of acute illness, the airway may become compromised for a variety of reasons and the lungs can fail to function. Both of these problems can result in either inadequate or absent breathing, each of which represents a highly undesirable situation. Health professionals must be able to recognise problems with the airway and breathing and then respond to these by providing appropriate escalating care. As well as this reactive approach, health professionals should endeavour to identify those patients who are at risk of a developing respiratory problem and take action to prevent its occurrence, or if this is not possible then measures should be instigated that enable a problem to be recognised early.

To understand the problems that can occur with the airway and breathing it is necessary to first hold a robust understanding of the anatomy of the upper airway and the respiratory system that it feeds. Only when this knowledge is firmly established will it be possible to understand how problems with the airway and breathing can develop and how these are managed. In this chapter these topics will be addressed in the same logical order: first the anatomy of the respiratory system will be outlined; then the common problems that can occur with the airway and breathing will be explained; and finally management options will be appraised.

Anatomy and physiology of the respiratory system

The anatomy and physiology of the respiratory system, which is pertinent to the care of those who are acutely ill, can be summarised through examining four anatomical areas. These are:

- The head and neck (see cross-section in Figure 4.1)
- The structures of the larynx (Figure 4.2)
- The thoracic cavity (Figure 4.3)
- The blood–air interface (Figure 4.4).

Once one is familiar with the structures that make up the respiratory system, it is possible to understand the physiology that underpins the mechanisms of breathing and the gas exchange that takes place between the body and the atmosphere. Again, once these basic principles are clearly understood, it should be easy to appreciate how insults to the structures of the respiratory system can inhibit respiratory function, resulting in an airway or breathing problem.

The airway is the path that air takes from the atmosphere through the mouth and nose via neck and into the lungs. For breathing to be effective the airway must be constantly kept clear (patent). Figure 4.1 shows a cross-section of the head and neck. From this view it is possible to identify the structures that make up the upper airway and the route that the airway takes to the trachea. Understanding this diagram will help appreciation of how the upper airway can become obstructed, how basic airway manoeuvres work to open the airway and how airway devices are inserted.

Figure 4.2 shows the structures of the larynx. The larynx, or voice box, separates the upper airway from the lower airway. To protect the lower airway from contamination, the larynx implements a number of mechanisms that help to keep the lower airway free from inhaled solids or liquids.

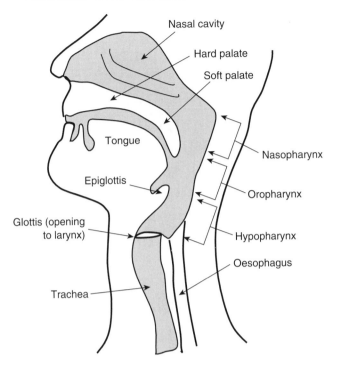

FIGURE 4.1   *Cross-section of the head and neck.*

Knowledge of laryngeal anatomy is important in understanding not only the function of these protective mechanisms, but also how some of the advanced airway manoeuvres contribute to securing the airway. For example, tracheal intubation involves passing a tube directly into the trachea via the larynx. When the upper airway is totally blocked and tracheal intubation is not possible, a surgical airway can be created artificially by making a cut into the larynx.

The mechanisms of breathing

Figures 4.1 and 4.2 deal mainly with developing anatomical understanding of the upper airway. They do little though to explain how breathing takes place and how gas is exchanged. Breathing is a two-stage process which consists of ventilation of the lungs and oxygenation of the blood. Ventilation is the movement of air in and out of the lungs, while oxygenation is the exchange of gases between the atmosphere and the blood. For respiration to function normally both stages must take place in a synergistic relationship.

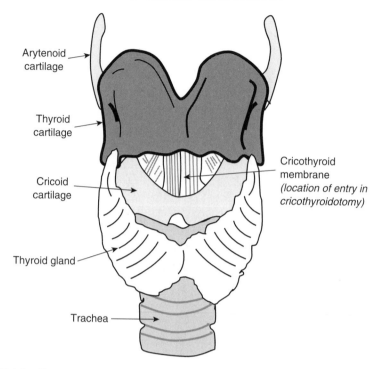

Arytenoid cartilage

Thyroid cartilage

Cricoid cartilage

Cricothyroid membrane
(location of entry in cricothyroidotomy)

Thyroid gland

Trachea

FIGURE 4.2   *The structures of the larynx.*

Ventilation

Figure 4.3 shows the structures of the respiratory system and how these are located within the thoracic cavity (chest). An understanding of this diagram is needed in order to understand how ventilation takes place. During ventilation air is moved in and out of the lungs via the airways. Pressure changes occur in the thoracic cavity resulting in a movement of air. To move air into the lungs (inhalation) the diaphragm contracts and flattens, the intercostal muscles may also contract, lifting the rib cage upwards and outwards. Both of these actions have the effect of increasing the amount of space in the chest, in turn creating a negative pressure (suction) in the chest which draws air into the lungs from the atmosphere. To breathe out (exhale) the reverse occurs: the diaphragm relaxes and returns to its resting dome shape. At the same time, any contraction of the intercostal muscles is reversed, causing the ribs to move inwards and downwards. Together these events reduce the size of the chest and create a positive pressure within the chest, resulting in air being forced out via the airway.

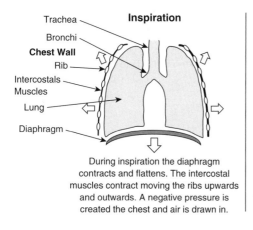
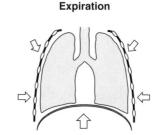

Inspiration	Expiration

Trachea
Bronchi
Chest Wall
Rib
Intercostals Muscles
Lung
Diaphragm

During inspiration the diaphragm contracts and flattens. The intercostal muscles contract moving the ribs upwards and outwards. A negative pressure is created the chest and air is drawn in.

During expiration the diaphragm relaxes and becomes dome shaped. The intercostal muscles relax allowing the ribs to move downwards and inwards. A positive pressure is created the chest and air is forced out.

FIGURE 4.3 *The thoracic cavity and mechanisms of breathing.*

Movement of the chest wall alone is not sufficient to bring about ventilation of the lungs. For the lungs to be ventilated they must be attached to the chest wall so that movement of the chest wall brings about expansion and compression of the lungs. The lungs are attached to the chest wall by the pleura, a double-layered fibrous membrane that is continuous with itself. The outer layer of the pleura is referred to as the parietal layer and this is firmly attached to the chest wall. The inner or visceral layer is firmly adhered to the outer surface of the lungs. The two layers of pleura are not formally attached to each other though in health they are held in close apposition. This is achieved by the presence of a small amount of pleural fluid in the space between the two pleural layers. The pleural fluid not only serves to keep the two layers of pleura together, but it also acts as a lubricant facilitating the expansion and contraction of the lungs. The lungs themselves are elastic structures that easily stretch and recoil with movements of the chest wall, much like an elastic band which can stretch and return to its original shape. This mechanism allows air both to enter the expanded lungs and to leave the relaxed lungs with ease.

Oxygenation

Having established how the lungs are ventilated, the next stage is to consider how oxygenation, the process of taking oxygen from the air in the lungs and passing it into the blood takes place. The body's ability to

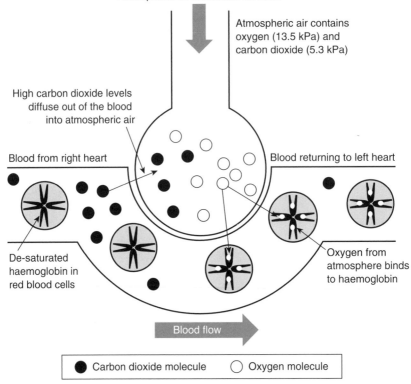

Atmospheric air drawn into alveolus

Atmospheric air contains
oxygen (13.5 kPa) and
carbon dioxide (5.3 kPa)

High carbon dioxide levels
diffuse out of the blood
into atmospheric air

Blood from right heart

Blood returning to left heart

De-saturated
haemoglobin in
red blood cells

Oxygen from
atmosphere binds
to haemoglobin

Blood flow

● Carbon dioxide molecule   ○ Oxygen molecule

FIGURE 4.4   *The blood–air interface in a healthy lung. Blood with high levels of carbon dioxide and low levels of oxygen enters the lungs. Carbon dioxide diffuses out of the blood and oxygen binds to haemoglobin in the red blood cells. The blood is then ready to be recirculated around the body.*

oxygenate blood is dependent on the ability to bring air rich in oxygen into close proximity with blood and for diffusion of gases to take place. Gas exchange takes place in the functional units of the lung called acini (singular, acinus). Each acinus consists of a group of alveoli and the respiratory bronchiole. Figure 4.4 shows how in the alveoli blood is brought into close contact with air. Here the process of diffusion is brought into effect. Diffusion works on the principle that a chemical present at different concentrations will move along the concentration gradient, from an area of higher concentration to an area of lower concentration. The principle of gas diffusion is dependent on partial pressure.

The concept of partial pressure is helpful when understanding how gases diffuse into a fluid. The partial pressure of a gas represents the contribution of one individual gas within a mixture of gases to the total pressure of that gas mixture. If other gases were removed the pressure of the gas remaining would be equal to the original partial pressure of the gas. Gases move from an area of high pressure to an area of low pressure.

Blood that is returned to the lungs after circulating around the body contains low levels (concentrations/partial pressure) of oxygen and high levels of carbon dioxide. This blood is classed as deoxygenated. When the chemical composition of deoxygenated blood is compared with that of the air which is drawn into the lungs during ventilation, deoxygenated blood contains higher levels of carbon dioxide and lower levels of oxygen than the air in the lungs. This puts in place a concentration gradient which allows diffusion of gases, both into and out of the blood, with carbon dioxide leaving the blood and oxygen entering the blood. These changes convert deoxygenated blood into oxygenated blood making it ready for recirculation around the body.

In the above brief sections on respiratory anatomy and physiology, some basic principles have been introduced, specifically those needed to understand the normal function of the respiratory system. Before reading on, you are strongly advised to ensure that you are familiar with the location and function of all of the structures that are shown in Figures 4.1–4.4. Doing this will help to ensure that you can make sense of the remainder of this chapter. To augment the information provided you may also wish to spend some time with an anatomy textbook in order to deepen your knowledge to a level that has not been possible here.

Problems with the airway and breathing

Airway and breathing problems originate from an inability of the lungs to either ventilate or oxygenate. Some patients will have problems that affect both ventilation and oxygenation at the same time. Occasionally, these problems have a single cause such as an airway obstruction which will both prevent ventilation and oxygenation due to the lack of air in the lungs. It is also possible for an individual patient to have two unrelated problems that affect both oxygenation and ventilation. Infective exacerbation of chronic obstructive pulmonary disease (COPD) is one such example. In COPD, the person has a chronic lung disease that causes ventilation problems and some oxygenation problems. If infection is added into the equation, inflammatory exudates are secreted into the lungs, further inhibiting oxygenation. While there are many causes of ventilation and oxygenation problems, some of the core causes are summarised in Box 4.1.

BOX 4.1 Common problems affecting the ability of the lungs to ventilate and oxygenate

Ventilation failure

- *Airway obstruction (Physical obstruction to normal air movement)*

    o Flaccid tongue and epiglottis
    o Vomit
    o Secretions
    o Food and other foreign objects
    o Blood
    o Swelling of the airways
    o Strangulation
    o Changed anatomy via trauma
    o Inhalation burns
    o Asthma (inflamed airways limit airflow)
    o COPD (flaccid airways trap air in the lungs on expiration)
    o Intraluminal tumour growth

- *Neuromuscular dysfunction (failure of the nerves or muscles needed to move the chest wall or diaphragm)*

    o Motor neurone disease
    o Muscular dystrophy
    o Head/neck injury
    o Stroke

- *Chest wall and airway integrity (prevents chest expansion)*

    o Burns to chest wall
    o Crush injuries
    o Multiple rib fractures
    o Ruptured trachea/bronchus

- *Pleural space injury (separates lung from chest wall preventing full expansion of the lung)*

    o Pneumothorax
    o Haemothorax
    o Pleural effusion

Oxygenation failure

- *Physiological shunting in the lungs (blood passes through the lungs without being exposed to oxygen)*

  o Consolidation
  o Collapse of alveoli (atelectasis)
  o Ventilation of the lungs with atmospheric air that has a low oxygen content

- *Ventilation perfusion mismatch*

  o Blood directed to areas of lung that is not well ventilated
  o Blood not directed to the lungs; pulmonary embolism; septal defect in the heart with right-to-left shunt of blood

- *Blood disorders (blood not able to take up oxygen)*

  o Reduced haemoglobin in the blood (anaemia)
  o Haemoglobin already saturated with another gas such as in carbon monoxide poisoning
  o Diseases of haemoglobin

Respiratory failure and tissue hypoxia

When a ventilation or oxygenation problem starts to upset homeostatic balance, respiratory failure is said to have occurred. Respiratory failure is defined as a level of oxygen in the blood of less than 8 kPa. There are two types of respiratory failure:

- **Type 1 respiratory failure** is as a result of low levels of oxygen in the blood. Type 1 respiratory failure is also known as hypoxaemic respiratory failure.
- **Type 2 respiratory failure** is characterised by low levels of oxygen in the blood (hypoxaemia) with the addition of an increase in the level of carbon dioxide in the blood (6 kPa or greater). Type 2 respiratory failure is also known as hypercapnic respiratory failure.

To understand the mechanisms that lead to the development of respiratory failure, it is helpful to consider how gas is transported in the blood. While some oxygen is carried dissolved in the blood, the majority of oxygen is transported in the blood bound to the haemoglobin found in the red blood cells. Each molecule of haemoglobin is only able to carry so much oxygen before it is fully saturated. The saturation of haemoglobin with oxygen is dependent on haemoglobin being exposed to oxygen in the lungs and the haemoglobin being available to accept oxygen. Where there is a deficiency of haemoglobin, or the haemoglobin is diseased, or oxygen is not available to the haemoglobin then the oxygen content of the blood will be reduced.

Carbon dioxide, the acidic waste product of respiration, is carried to the lungs dissolved in blood plasma. As the transport of carbon dioxide is not dependent on the presence of functional haemoglobin, excretion of carbon dioxide can be increased by increasing ventilation of the lungs. It is this difference in how oxygen and carbon dioxide are transported that accounts for the development of either type 1 (hypoxaemic) or type 2 (hypercapnic) respiratory failure.

Figure 4.5 shows how some of the blood that passes through the lungs fails to reach well-ventilated alveoli. Blood that passes poorly ventilated alveoli will not be able to give up the high levels of carbon dioxide that it contains or take on additional supplies of oxygen. The result of this is that blood is recirculated around the body with a lower level of oxygen and a higher level of carbon dioxide than normal (Figure 4.5). Blood that passed poorly ventilated alveoli is mixed with the blood that passed well-ventilated alveoli as it is circulated around the body. To compensate for this slight disarrangement, the lungs attempt to increase ventilation. This attempt to increase ventilation causes one of four things to occur:

- The person recruits more fully functional lung and ventilates it as normal (breathes more deeply)
- The person ventilates the lung tissue more rapidly, without increasing the amount of lung involved in breathing
- The person breathes more deeply and more rapidly (recruiting more lung and ventilating it more often)
- The person is unable to initiate or sustain increased ventilation.

Normal breathing uses only a small portion of the lungs. If part of this portion is diseased or poorly ventilated the body attempts to recruit additional healthy lung. This is achieved by the person taking deeper breaths. This response is similar to what happens when a person exercises and the body needs more oxygen. In exercise the respiratory rate and depth increase to address the body's additional demands for oxygen and the need to excrete higher levels of carbon dioxide. At times of illness, breathing more deeply increases the amount of functional lung involved in oxygenation and aims to compensate for the respiratory problem, restoring normal homeostatic balance. An alternative to recruiting more lung tissue is to ventilate the lungs more rapidly without increasing the depth of inspiration. This is a less than ideal situation as it means that diseased,

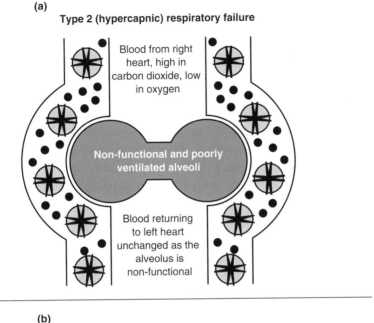

(a)

Type 2 (hypercapnic) respiratory failure

Blood from right heart, high in carbon dioxide, low in oxygen

Non-functional and poorly ventilated alveoli

Blood returning to left heart unchanged as the alveolus is non-functional

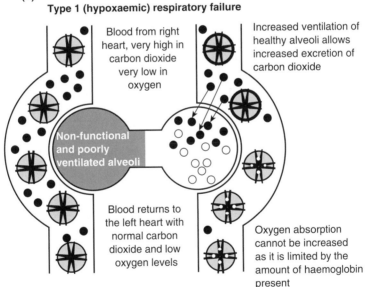

(b)

Type 1 (hypoxaemic) respiratory failure

Blood from right heart, very high in carbon dioxide very low in oxygen

Increased ventilation of healthy alveoli allows increased excretion of carbon dioxide

Non-functional and poorly ventilated alveoli

Blood returns to the left heart with normal carbon dioxide and low oxygen levels

Oxygen absorption cannot be increased as it is limited by the amount of haemoglobin present

FIGURE 4.5   *Mechanisms leading to respiratory failure. (a) Type 2 hypercapnic, (b) type 1 hypoxaemic.*

non-functional lung tissue will still receive blood and this blood will leave the lungs without taking up sufficient oxygen or giving out the carbon dioxide that it contains.

Where a significant amount of lung disease exists, differences in the way that oxygen and carbon dioxide are carried in the blood give rise to the development of either type 1 hypoxaemic or type 2 hypercapnic respiratory failure. Figure 4.5 shows how when the blood passes non-functional lung tissue it takes up no additional oxygen. Essentially, it is shunted through the lungs. Likewise, carbon dioxide in the blood cannot be excreted into non-functional lung. When the shunted blood is mixed with blood which has passed healthy, well-ventilated lung the result is blood with an oxygen content which is less than normal and a carbon dioxide level that is slightly higher than normal. When this blood is recirculated through the lungs, one of two outcomes can occur depending on how the body is able to compensate.

The slightly increased amount of carbon dioxide in the blood causes an increase in the concentration gradient between the carbon dioxide level in blood and the air contained in the well-ventilated alveoli (Figure 4.5b). If some blood is directed to well-ventilated alveoli, an increased amount of carbon dioxide can be excreted at this location, returning the carbon dioxide level of the blood to normal. This remains true even if a proportion of the blood is directed to diseased or poorly ventilated alveoli. This prevents the development of hypercapnia. If, however, all the blood returned to the lungs is directed to diseased, poorly ventilated alveoli, extra carbon dioxide cannot be expelled and the carbon dioxide level of the blood will increase progressively until hypercapnia develops (Figure 4.5a). The increased excretion of carbon dioxide in functional lung is possible because carbon dioxide is carried to the lungs freely dissolved in plasma. This makes its excretion solely dependent on the presence of a concentration gradient.

Unfortunately, this same compensation is not possible for oxygen take-up in the lungs. You will recall that for oxygen to be transported in the blood it must be bound to haemoglobin. Each molecule of haemoglobin is only able to carry a finite amount of oxygen. Once the haemoglobin is saturated with oxygen it is not able to carry any additional oxygen. It follows therefore that blood passing the functional alveoli will become fully saturated with oxygen yet the blood passing the poorly ventilated alveoli will not. Once these two types of blood are mixed on return to the heart the result is blood with a lower level of oxygen than is normal. How severe the respiratory failure will become will depend on how much lung is functional and diseased. The need for oxygen to be bound to haemoglobin explains how type 1 respiratory failure develops (Figure 4.5b).

While the above explanations of the mechanism of respiratory failure explain the condition in simple terms, they do tend to compartmentalise the different types of respiratory failure. A word of caution is needed in order to avoid missing an important pathological change – the starting point in doing this is to recognise that respiratory failure is a complex and dynamic condition. For some, respiratory failure will be an acute event, while for others respiratory failure will be a chronic state. In both the acute and chronic stages of respiratory failure people can move from type 1 to type 2 respiratory failure relatively rapidly and this is something of which those involved in the care of the acutely ill must be aware. To illustrate the dynamic nature of respiratory failure both in the acute and chronic stages it is useful to consider the changes that can occur during acute asthma and infective exacerbation of COPD.

In the early stages of an acute asthma attack, a person experiences a ventilation problem to a portion of the lung. To counter this, the patient can increase ventilation to non-inflamed areas of the lungs. If the inflammation of the airways is not quickly resolved or it progresses rapidly then the patient can soon tire of ventilating additional lung fields or become unable to ventilate lungs with widespread inflammation. This can result in the person quickly moving from type 1 respiratory failure to type 2 respiratory failure.

A similar situation can occur in patients with COPD. Here patients have a problem with ventilating their lungs that results in air becoming trapped in parts of the lung. This essentially renders the part of the lung with trapped air as non-functional, causing a physiological shunt, which can result in chronic respiratory failure. To combat this problem people with COPD utilise the reserve capacity in the lungs during normal day-to-day breathing. If an acute infection is added to this chronic lung problem then, given that reserve capacity is already in day-to-day use, there is little additional reserve capacity available to compensate for the infection. This can cause the person to experience a worsening of their respiratory problem and they may develop a second acute type of respiratory failure on top of their chronic condition.

While respiratory failure is a problem with lung function, the sequel of respiratory failure has widespread implications for the maintenance of homeostasis and the body as a whole. Hypercapnic respiratory failure has the effect of altering the pH of the body, making the body fluids more acidic. Hypoxaemic respiratory failure limits the amount of oxygen available to the cells of the body resulting in cell injury and death. When the oxygen supply to the cells of the body is reduced, a condition called 'tissue hypoxia' develops. There are a number of causes of tissue hypoxia and not all are respiratory in origin; in fact, only one of the four causes of tissue hypoxia is respiratory. It makes sense, however, to mention the other causes of tissue hypoxia at this stage even though they are mainly circulatory in origin. Thus the causes of tissue hypoxia can be summarised as:

- A lack of oxygen in the blood (hypoxaemia, principally a respiratory problem)
- Poor circulation (stagnant and ischaemic hypoxia)
- Lack of red blood cells to carry oxygen to the tissues (anaemic hypoxia)
- Inability of the oxygen in the blood to be used by the tissues (histotoxic hypoxia).

In a respiratory context, assessing for the presence of hypoxaemia is of paramount importance. This is achieved by a combination of pulse oximetry and arterial blood gas analysis.

Supporting the airway and breathing

Having read this far, you should now be clear that respiratory problems result from a problem either with ventilating the lung or oxygenating the blood. To solve respiratory problems, therefore, health professionals must ensure that the lungs can ventilate correctly and that gas exchange takes place in the lungs. In practical terms this equates with the patient having clear airways through which the lungs can be ventilated and that air rich in oxygen is brought into close contact with blood in healthy alveoli. The remainder of this chapter will deal with resolving the problems that arise from a failure of ventilation or oxygenation.

Recognising airway problems and securing the airway

Airway problems occur frequently in those who are acutely ill. Recognising and treating airway problems must be a priority for all health professionals as an obstructed airway will have a serious and detrimental impact on the person's ability to ventilate and oxygenate. Airway obstructions can be classified as complete or partial and some example causes of airway obstruction were listed in Box 4.1. Traditionally, when discussions of airway patency occur, they focus on the assessment and management of the upper airway. While this is pertinent, as upper airway problems are a common cause of airway obstruction, it is essential not to forget that airway problems can occur in the lower airway as a result of an inhaled foreign object, inflammation in the airway or damage to the airway, such as in COPD or the growth of a tumour into the airway. Recognition of an airway obstruction requires you to:

- Look
- Listen
- Feel

for evidence of an airway obstruction.

Look initially at the person to identify if they have any obvious signs of an airway obstruction or clear risk factors for developing an airway problem. Any person who is unconscious or who has a reduced level of consciousness has the potential to develop an airway problem and you should instigate airway care in this group of patients as a priority. Look to see if there is any evidence that the person may have had a cerebrovascular accident (stroke) or transient ischaemic attack as these conditions can result in the person loosing the protective gag reflex which helps to maintain a clear airway. Look also to see if there is any swelling of the airway or if there is a physical obstruction to the airway such as vomit or secretions. Look at the chest to see if it is expanding normally or if there is any evidence of see-saw breathing – a phenomenon that occurs when the airway is totally blocked yet the person is trying to breathe against the obstruction. A person who is choking is likely to be in obvious distress and they may clutch the throat.

At the same time as you are looking at the person, listen for any signs of airway obstruction. You should listen specifically for breath sounds and the presence of any added sounds. The quality of the person's voice and the inability to complete full sentences without taking a breath are important signs of a partial airway obstruction. Noisy breathing, such as breathing that has a grunting, snoring, bubbling or wheezing quality, indicates an airway obstruction. Stridor, a characteristic inspiratory wheeze that is created in the larger airway is always a sign of airway obstruction and warrants immediate assessment.

Finally, feel for any evidence of airway obstruction. Place you, cheek close to the person's open mouth and feel for the person's breath on your cheek, looking at the same time for movements of the chest. This is a test to see if there is normal airflow and must be performed with a basic airway manoeuvre such as the head tilt-chin lift described later in this chapter. It is only a valuable test in people who are unconscious, as people who are able to talk or cough have some degree of airflow, even if it is not normal.

When an airway problem is identified there are several techniques that can be used to relieve the obstruction. These range from the simple adjustment of a person's posture to more complicated procedures that require surgical skill. Airway management should start with basic manoeuvres as these techniques are often sufficient to open the airway. Where basic manoeuvres fail to secure the airway or there are specific risks to the airway then more advanced methods should be employed. Some of the commonly performed airway manoeuvres are listed in Box 4.2. The role of each of these procedures is discussed in turn below.

BOX 4.2   Airway management techniques

Upper airway

- Basic airway manoeuvres

  - Head tilt-chin lift
  - Jaw thrust
  - Recovery position
  - Back slaps
  - Abdominal thrusts
  - Chest thrusts

- Simple airway adjuncts

  - Suction
  - Oropharyngeal airway
  - Nasopharyngeal airway

- Intermediate airway devices

  - Laryngeal mask airway
  - Laryngeal tube
  - Combitube

- Advanced airway techniques

  - Tracheal intubation
  - Cricothyroidotomy

Lower airways

- Bronchodilators
- Steroids

The basic airway manoeuvres

Basic airway manoeuvres are those techniques that can be performed without any specialist equipment. They represent the starting point of all airway care although they are often poorly performed or neglected in favour of more advanced techniques. Failure to perform basic airway care correctly has been highlighted as a reason for increased mortality in those who become acutely ill, and the utility of these techniques should not be underestimated. The basic techniques can be divided into those manoeuvres that should be used to protect the airway in all semiconscious or unconscious patients and those manoeuvres that are specifically directed at relieving total airway obstruction or choking.

The most important airway manoeuvre is that of the head tilt–chin lift. When a person loses consciousness the airway becomes more flaccid. This can result in the structures of the airway falling against each other and obstructing the flow of air. Placing one palm on the person's forehead and two fingers under the chin, tilting the head back and lifting the chin up is usually successful in separating the flaccid structures and provides space for air to pass (Figure 4.6a).

An alternative method for opening the airway is the jaw thrust. This technique is slightly more difficult to perform and is usually reserved for use in cases of trauma where there is suspicion of injury to the cervical spine. The jaw thrust is useful in these circumstances as it can open the airway without moving the neck. This reduces the risk of worsening any cervical injury that may be present. To perform jaw thrust you need to be at the head of the patient. Place your fingers behind the angle of the jaw and your thumbs on the chin. Next lift the jaw upwards and push the chin down with your thumbs. This will usually clear the airway by separating flaccid airway structures. Figure 4.6b illustrates how the jaw thrust is performed.

While the above two techniques are very helpful in opening an airway that has become obstructed by flaccid airway structures, they are of little use when it comes to dealing with a build-up of liquids in the airway or the presence of solid matter. When lying on the back any airway secretions, regurgitated stomach contents or blood will collect at the back of the throat and obstruct the airway. These secretions may also be inhaled into the lungs where they can precipitate pneumonia, which will complicate the person's recovery. To avoid these problems in the spontaneously breathing patient the recovery position should be used to allow any fluid to drain from the airway.

Although many different recovery positions have been described over the years, important features of any recovery position have been identified by the European Resuscitation Council (Handley et al., 2005). It acknowledges that any recovery position should:

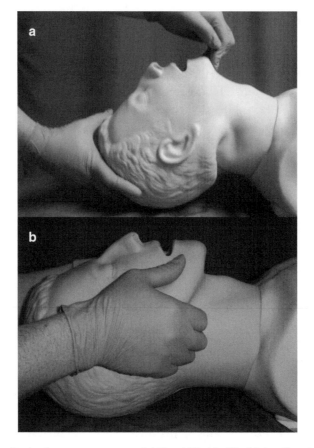

FIGURE 4.6   *Basic airway manoeuvres. (a) Head tilt-chin lift, (b) Jaw thrust.*

- Be stable
- As close to true lateral position as possible
- The head should be dependent (angled downwards)
- No pressure should be put on the chest, which could impair breathing.

Complying with these features will ensure that the person is as safe as possible.

Foreign body airway obstruction

A number of foreign bodies can obstruct the airway. By far the most common of these is food, though many other objects have been reported to cause airway compromise. When this occurs the person is said to have choked. Choking can result in total or partial airway obstruction. Each of these requires a separate approach to its management. If the airway obstruction is partial, the person should still be able to cough effectively. Coughing is by far the most helpful way of clearing the airway. If a patient is conscious and has an effective cough then they should be encouraged to cough, as this will often be successful in clearing the airway. If the person is not able to cough or tires of coughing, then further action is needed to secure the airway. Further interventions are centred on cycles of back slaps and abdominal thrusts for the conscious patient or cardiopulmonary resuscitation (CPR) for the person who has become unconscious.

Back slaps are performed on the conscious patient when coughing has failed to clear the obstruction and the person's cough has become ineffective or when the person never had an effective cough. To perform back slaps, stand at the side of the person, leaning them well forward. Place one hand so that it supports the chest. Then with your other hand administer up to five sharp back slaps with the heel of your hand, in between the shoulder blades. After each back slap check to see if the airway has been cleared. If the airway is cleared you do not need to continue to administer all five back slaps.

If after giving five back slaps the airway is not cleared the next step is to administer up to five abdominal thrusts. To do this stand behind the person, lean them well forward and place both your arms around the upper abdomen. With one hand make a fist and with the other hand grasp the clenched fist and place your hands in the space created between the base of the breast bone and the umbilicus. Then pull inwards and upwards up to five times. After each thrust, check to see if the airway has cleared. If after five abdominal thrusts the airway is not cleared repeat five back slaps, then continue to alternate sets of five back slaps with five abdominal thrusts until the airway is cleared. If the person should lose consciousness then immediately call for help and start CPR. Any person who has had abdominal thrusts performed upon them or who has continuing symptoms should be examined by a doctor.

Abdominal thrusts may be impossible in some groups of patients, such as those who are obese, and dangerous in others, such as those who are pregnant. Chest thrusts present an alternative to abdominal thrusts in these situations. To perform chest thrusts the arms are placed around the chest instead of the abdomen. An inward force is then applied to the chest wall up to five times, again checking after each thrust to see if the airway obstruction has been relieved.

If the above first aid methods fail to remove the object, the situation is quite serious. Those who have received advanced training may use a laryngoscope and attempt to directly visualise the offending object and if possible remove it using Magill's forceps (see Figure 4.8). If this is not possible then a cricothyroidotomy may become necessary – these procedures are described later in the section on advanced airway procedures.

Simple airway adjuncts

Simple airway adjuncts, such as the oropharyngeal airway (OPA) and nasopharyngeal airway (NPA) are useful additions to the basic airway manoeuvres and can be safely used by health professionals to provide improved airway care. It must be recognised that these devices need to be used in conjunction with basic airway manoeuvres if optimal airway care is to be provided. These airway devices only support the structures of the upper airway and do little to protect the airway from secretions or vomit. Suction can be used as an adjunct to remove vomit and secretions from the airway.

The OPA (Figure 4.7a) is the first-line airway device employed by many and is by far the most commonly used device out of the two simple

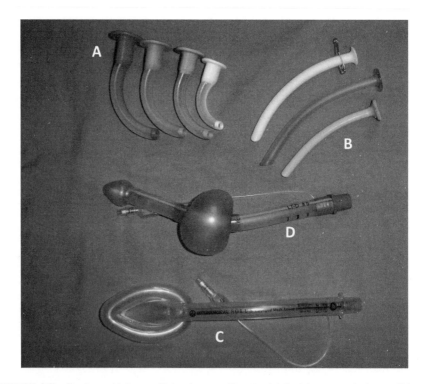

FIGURE 4.7   *Basic and intermediate airway adjuncts. (a) Oropharyngeal airway, (b) nasopharyngeal airway, (c) laryngeal mask airway, (d) laryngeal tube.*

airway devices available. OPAs can only be used in patients who are sufficiently unconscious to have lost their gag reflex – the protective involuntary reflex that helps to expel foreign objects that enter the airway. Using an OPA in a person who has an intact gag reflex can cause retching, which can lead to vomiting, in turn further threatening the airway. Retching can also lead to a raised intracranial pressure, which can worsen the condition of any patient who has a head injury or other intracranial pathology, such as a bleed or embolism, and will precipitate movement of the neck, which can worsen cervical spinal injuries when present. Ensuring the patient is sufficiently unconscious to receive an OPA is a mandatory consideration.

To be effective, the correct size OPA must be used. Airways that are too long can impinge on the epiglottis and risk causing laryngospasm, a closure of the larynx which can potentially be fatal. An OPA that is too small will fall short of where it is intended to sit and will do more to block the airway than assist in maintaining it. To identify the correct size of an OPA for a patient, place the airway by the patient's incisors. The correct size will extend to the angle of the jaw. In general, size 2 (green) OPAs are suitable for small adults; size 3 (orange) being for average adults; and size 4 (red) most suited to large adults. The procedure for insertion of an OPA is described in Box 4.3.

BOX 4.3 Insertion procedure for an OPA

1 Ensure that the patient is unresponsive before attempting to insert an OPA
2 Ensure that you have the correct size of OPA
3 Inspect the mouth for any foreign objects, remove if present
4 Perform head tilt-chin lift and open the patient's mouth
5 Invert the airway
6 Insert the airway into the mouth half its length
7 Rotate the airway while continuing to insert the remainder of its length until the bite block rests against the teeth
8 Check that air is flowing freely through the airway
9 Continue to support the airway with basic manoeuvres
10 Check the position and patency of the airway regularly

N.B.: If the patient starts to gag or retch at any point during the insertion, immediately remove the airway device. Do not attempt to reinsert it but resort to more basic airway manoeuvres to maintain the airway!

NPAs (Figure 4.7b) present a useful alternative to the OPA. Situations that are suited to NPA use include patients who have a clenched (trismus) jaw or patients who have an intact gag reflex but still require some airway support. The main advantage of the NPA over the OPA is that the NPA can be used in conscious individuals.

NPAs are less commonly used than OPAs; the reason for this is likely to be multi-faceted. Firstly, NPAs are slightly more difficult to insert than OPAs. Secondly, their use can precipitate nasal bleeding, compounding any airway problems. Like OPAs, the correct size of NPA must be selected. A 6-mm internal diameter tube is the usual size for an adult female and a 7-mm internal diameter is the standard choice for an adult male. The length of the tube is governed by the internal diameter, but tubes that are too long can precipitate laryngospasm. Caution must be exercised when using NPAs in small or short individuals.

Traditionally, a suspected or confirmed fractured base of skull was an absolute contraindication to the use of NPAs due to the risk of inserting the airway into the brain. More recent thinking now indicates that this is a rare complication and the risk of brain injury is less than the risks associated with airway obstruction. If there is no other alternative to using an NPA in a patient with a fractured base of skull then the NPA should be used to secure the airway despite the risk of brain injury. A contraindication to the use of NPAs would be a clotting or bleeding disorder, as bleeding often caused by insertion of the NPA may be difficult to control. To insert an NPA, follow the procedure outlined in Box 4.4.

BOX 4.4 Insertion procedure for an NPA

1 Select an appropriately sized NPA (adults: 6 mm females; 7 mm males)
2 Insert a safety pin through the flanged end of the airway if the device does not have an integral inhalation guard
3 Lubricate the airway with a water-based lubricant such as KY Jelly
4 Insert the airway into the right nostril up to the flange
5 If resistance is encountered, remove the airway and attempt to insert the airway into the left nostril
6 Once successfully inserted, check that:

   ○ Air is flowing through the airway
   ○ The airway is visible in the back of the throat
   ○ Bleeding is not caused by the insertion of the airway

N.B.: If airflow through a single NPA is inadequate, bilateral placement can increase airflow.

Intermediate airway devices

While the simple airway adjuncts are useful in supporting the soft tissues of the airway, they do little to protect the airway from secretions, vomit or blood. Traditionally, the only way that this level of protection could be achieved was through the use of tracheal intubation and this still remains the gold standard for airway care. Tracheal intubation, however, is a difficult skill to learn and requires substantial practice. As such, it is not a skill that can be taught to, or maintained by, large numbers of health professionals. Developments in technology have seen the advent of the intermediate airway devices which are relatively simple to use and offer a number of benefits over the OPA and NPA. Coupled with this, research evidence has demonstrated that these intermediate devices can be used safely and effectively by health professionals in the management of the acutely ill and particularly those requiring resuscitation.

Intermediate airways are longer than the simple airways and are passed further into the patient's throat. This takes them closer to the glottis, the opening to the larynx and the lower airway. This, combined with the inflatable cuffs that are a feature of many of the intermediate airway devices, enables them to provide improved protection of the airway from secretions, blood and vomit when compared to the OPA and NPA. A further benefit of the intermediate airway devices is that when used during cardiac arrest, chest compressions need not be interrupted to facilitate their insertion and ventilation may be possible, again without interrupting chest compressions, although further research is needed to confirm this.

Several intermediate airway devices have been invented and used to a greater or lesser degree. Those devices that have achieved popularity will be discussed here: the laryngeal mask (Figure 4.7c) and the laryngeal tube (LT) (Figure 4.7d).

Laryngeal Mask

The laryngeal mask airway (LMA) consists of a semi-rigid tube with a spoon-shaped attachment. This spoon-shaped attachment is bordered with a cuff that is inflated to form a seal over the opening to the larynx, thus protecting the airway. In the UK, the LMA is the most widely accepted intermediate airway device and much experience has been gained in its use, both during anaesthesia and resuscitation.

The principal indication for the LMA is when an unconscious person requires ventilation. The technique of ventilating a person through a LMA is thought to be easier than using a bag and mask device and it is less likely to cause regurgitation of gastric contents or result in aspiration when compared to bag and mask ventilation. The European Resuscitation Council recommends (Nolan et al. 2005) that where an LMA can be inserted without delay, bag and mask ventilation should be avoided altogether, favouring the immediate insertion of an LMA and ventilating using a bag via this route. Despite the benefits of the LMA, there are some disadvantages of the device that are noteworthy. Firstly, some patients cannot be successfully ventilated using the LMA. It is possible that LMAs are associated with a higher risk of pulmonary aspiration of gastric contents than is seen with tracheal intubation. The risk of aspiration is higher still with OPAs and NPAs, and the LMA presents a compromise position. The procedure used to insert an LMA is outlined in Box 4.5.

BOX 4.5 Procedure for insertion of an LMA

1 Select the appropriately sized device (small adults size 4; large adults size 5)
2 Check the integrity of the cuff by inflating it with the stated volume of air
3 Deflate the cuff fully against a clean flat surface or gloved palm
4 Ensure a syringe is available, drawn up with the correct volume of air needed to inflate the cuff
5 Lubricate the posterior aspect of the airway only with water-soluble lubricant
6 Apply head tilt-chin lift manoeuvre if no spinal injury is suspected
7 Hold the LMA with the open end facing towards the patient's feet and your first finger behind the mask extended along the tube
8 Insert the LMA into the patient's mouth
9 Push the LMA up against the hard palate and insert it into the person's throat until resistance is felt. Keeping the LMA pushed against the hard palate during insertion prevents inversion of the epiglottis, which can obstruct the airway
10 With your free hand hold the LMA in place and remove the hand which is in the mouth
11 Inflate the cuff with the required volume of air
12 Connect the LMA to the self-inflating bag via a catheter mount
13 Ventilate the patient and check to see that the chest rises symmetrically and that breath sounds can be heard bilaterally with a stethoscope
14 Secure the tube in place

Precautions

- Do not use force to insert the airway
- If resistance is felt, try repositioning the airway
- If gagging or retching occurs during insertion, immediately remove the device and resort to a more basic airway manoeuvre
- If the lungs cannot be immediately ventilated after insertion, remove the device and resort to more basic means

Laryngeal tube

The LT is a relatively new airway device, though it has quickly gained popularity, particularly for use in the out-of-hospital setting. Largely, the LT is a design improvement on the Combitube and some other older airway devices. In many centres the LT has replaced these devices. The LT consists of a single blind-ended tube with two cuffs that are inflated via a single inlet port. The smaller distal cuff obstructs the oesophagus and reduces the risk of regurgitation of gastric contents. The larger proximal cuff sits in the oropharynx and anchors the airway in place and reduces the risk of secretions from the upper airway entering the hypopharynx. Apertures in between the two cuffs sit opposite the glottis and allow the lungs to be ventilated. To date, experience with the LT is limited due to its novelty, and, while early evidence is good, further evidence is needed to confirm its place in the care of those who are acutely ill and particularly during resuscitation. One disadvantage of the LT is that it is contraindicated in patients who have oesophageal disease or those who have ingested caustic substances. To insert the LT follow the procedure outlined in Box 4.6.

BOX 4.6 Procedure for the insertion of the laryngeal tube

1 Select an appropriately sized LT (small adult 3, yellow; adult 4, red; large adult 5, purple)
2 Inflate the cuffs with the stated volumes of air to check cuff integrity
3 Deflate the cuffs
4 Lubricate the distal cuff and the bottom of the tube with a water-based lubricant. Do not lubricate the larger pharyngeal cuff or obstruct the apertures with lubricant
5 Open the person's mouth and lift the chin
6 Insert the airway in the midline and advance it so the mark shown on the tube is level with the teeth
7 Hold the tube in place and inflate the cuffs with the stated volume of air
8 Attach the self-inflating bag via a catheter mount and ventilate the patient
9 Ensure that the chest rises and that breath sounds can be heard on both sides of the chest

Precautions

- Do not use force to insert the airway
- If resistance is felt try repositioning the airway
- If gagging or retching occurs during insertion immediately remove the device and resort to a more basic airway manoeuvre
- If the lungs cannot be immediately ventilated after insertion remove the device and resort to more basic means

Advanced airway techniques

In the vast majority of circumstances and certainly in the initial management of those who are acutely ill, the basic manoeuvres and intermediate
airway devices are adequate to maintain the airway. In some circumstances,
and certainly as time progresses, more advanced airway care will be needed
by those who are acutely ill. Patients who require more advanced airway
care include those for whom:

- An airway cannot be obtained using more basic techniques
- The airway is at high risk from aspiration
- The airway is swollen or the anatomy is changed in some way
- A physical obstruction to the airway is present that cannot be removed.

When advanced airway care is required there are essentially two options:
tracheal intubation and, in extreme circumstances, cricothyroidotomy. As
has been alluded to previously, both of these techniques require extensive
skill and it is probable that most readers of this text will be assisting more
senior colleagues with performing these skills rather than performing them
independently. However, for patient care to be seamless, it is essential that
all those caring for people who may require advanced airway care are
familiar with these procedures so that more senior colleagues can be
assisted more efficiently.

Tracheal intubation

Tracheal intubation involves inserting a tube directly into the trachea with
the aid of a laryngoscope. The laryngoscope is an illuminated tool that is
used to both illuminate the airway and lift up the tongue so that the glottis
(the opening to the larynx and trachea) can be seen. A variety of laryngoscopes are now available, and not all are directly interchangeable, so check
that the equipment that you have is compatible. Most laryngoscopes come
in two distinct parts, the handle and the blade. The laryngoscope handle
(Figure 4.8, A) is the part that is held by the operator and connects to the
laryngoscope blade. The laryngoscope handle normally contains the power
source for the light, although there are some exceptions to this. Most han-
dles today have a hook-on connection to attach the blade. The laryngoscope blade is the aspect that is inserted into the patient's mouth and used
to displace and lift the tongue. Two main types of laryngoscope blade are
available on the market. These are Mackintosh (curved, Figure 4.8, B) and
Miller (straight, Figure 4.8, C). In the UK, Mackintosh blades are most

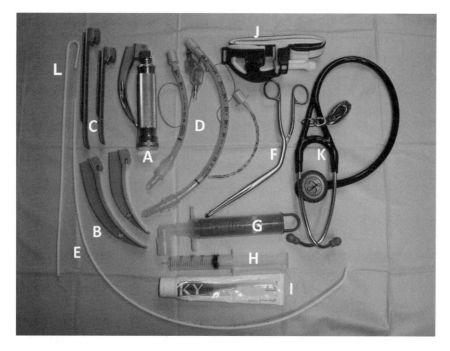

FIGURE 4.8   *Equipment used in tracheal intubation. A, laryngoscope handle (with blade mounted); B, Mackintosh blade; C, Miller blade; D, tracheal tubes with inflatable cuffs; E, gum elastic bougie; F, Magill's forceps; G, tube check device; H, syringe for cuff inflation; I, lubricant; J, tube tie; K, stethoscope to check tube placement; L, malleable stylet.*

commonly used for adults, while Miller blades are used for paediatric intubation.

Once the glottis has been viewed, the tracheal tube can be passed under direct vision into the trachea. In adults, the tracheal tube (Figure 4.8, D) has an inflatable cuff that isolates the airway and protects the trachea from the risk of aspiration. Intubation is a risky procedure and must only be undertaken by those who have demonstrated competency in the technique. Complications of intubation include damage to the teeth, inadvertent intubation of the oesophagus and pneumothorax. Intubation can precipitate cardiac arrest in certain individuals.

Successful intubation requires preparation and even in an emergency it is important to ensure that all the equipment required is available and functional so that it can be passed to the operator in a timely way. The procedure for preparation and intubation is outlined in Box 4.7.

BOX 4.7   Procedure for intubation

Gather and lay out equipment

- Appropriately sized tracheal tube (8 mm internal diameter is a universal adult size)
- Water-based lubricant
- Gauze
- Laryngoscope handle
- Laryngoscope blade of correct type and size 20-mL syringe
- Catheter mount
- Stethoscope
- Suction with a Yankauer tip switched on and close to hand
- Tube holder

1   Inflate the cuff on the tracheal tube to check its integrity then deflate it
2   Lubricate the distal part of the tube with water-based lubricant
3   Draw up 20 mL of air into the syringe
4   Attach the laryngoscope blade to the handle and check that it illuminates
5   Make a final check that all equipment is present and ready
6   Tell the person performing the intubation that you are ready to proceed.

Assist with intubation

1   Hand the laryngoscope to the person performing the intubation
2   Prepare to pass the tracheal tube when asked
3   Prepare to pass the syringe
4   Disconnect the mask from the self-inflating bag
5   Connect the catheter mount to the self-inflating bag
6   Prepare to pass the self-inflating bag
7   Prepare to pass the stethoscope
8   Prepare to pass the tube tie

While the procedure described in Box 4.7 outlines a simple technique, the use of gum elastic bougie (Figure 4.8, E) or malleable intubation stylets (Figure 4.8, L) may be used to aid the process. Bougies are passed into the trachea and then the tracheal tube is inserted over this device. The bougie aids intubation as it is narrower, thus allowing for better visualisation of the glottis. The malleable stylets are inserted into the tracheal tube prior to intubation. These make the tracheal tube more rigid so that it can be angled in a direction that assists with correct placement of the tube.

Cricothyroidotomy/cricothyroidotomy
Cricothyroidotomy is a procedure used to provide an airway in patients who cannot be ventilated or intubated. Cricothyroidotomy involves creating an

artificial opening into the neck to provide an airway when the normal airway is totally blocked. The opening is made through the cricothyroid membrane in the larynx. There are two options available to the practitioner – the use of either a needle or scalpel. The needle cricothyroidotomy is a short-term option and will only provide relief from an airway obstruction for around ten minutes. It does, though, require less skill to perform and may be sufficient to buy time until a definitive airway can be performed. A surgical airway performed with a scalpel will provide definitive relief for an airway obstruction. Like tracheal intubation, cricothyroidotomy is a more advanced skill and it is associated with complications such as damage to the vocal cords, bleeding and damage to the posterior laryngeal wall. Therefore, most readers of this text will be assisting with these procedures rather than performing them independently.

Needle cricothyroidotomy

Needle cricothyroidotomy essentially involves puncturing the cricothyroid membrane using a non-kinking cannula over needle. The needle is then removed and the cannula is attached to an oxygen source. The amount of oxygen that can be delivered through such a narrow bore cannula is limited and no expiration of gas is possible. These facts combined can lead to the development of barotrauma and/or carbon dioxide retention which explains why needle cricothyroidotomy is a procedure that can buy time only. A practical problem associated with needle cricothyroidotomy is kinking of the cannula with subsequent obstruction of the oxygen supply. As specialised kink-resistant cannulas are not widely available this is a problem that should be looked for, particularly if an intravenous cannula has been used to perform the procedure. Box 4.8 lists the equipment required to perform needle cricothyroidotomy.

BOX 4.8   Equipment needed to perform needle cricothyroidotomy

- 12- or 14-gauge cannula
- 10- or 20-mL syringe
- 3-way tap
- Oxygen tubing
- Oxygen supply running at 15 L/min

To prepare for a needle cricothyroidotomy, attach the syringe to the cannula and pass this to the operator performing the procedure. They

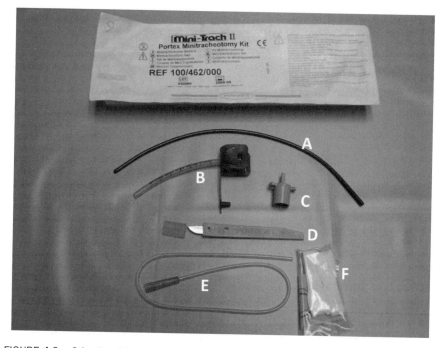

FIGURE 4.9   *Cricothyroidotomy Kit: Mini-Trach II. A, rigid introducer; B, mini tracheotomy tube; C, catheter mount; D, guarded scalpel; E, suction catheter; F, tube ties.*

will pierce the skin over the lower point of the cricoid membrane and then angle the needle towards the feet. Once in position the needle will be removed leaving the cannula in place. The 3-way tap is then attached to the oxygen supply with each of its pathways left open. This is then attached to the cannula. Jet ventilation is performed by placing a finger over the exhaust from the 3-way tap for one second and releasing it for a period of four seconds. This cycle is repeated until definitive care can be provided. If a 3-way tap is not available, a hole can be cut into oxygen tubing and this can be used in its place, being connected directly to the cannula.

Surgical airway

Commercially available kits exist for performing surgical cricothyroidotomy such as the Mini-Trach II (Figure 4.9) and PCK Portex cricothyroidotomy kit. However, an ordinary scalpel and a small tracheotomy tube will suffice if one of these kits is not available and the situation is an emergency. The benefit of using a kit such as the Mini-Trach II is that all of the equipment is contained in a convenient pack and the scalpel is guarded to help prevent injury to the posterior laryngeal wall.

The person performing the procedure will identify the landmarks in the neck and hold the skin taut prior to making the incision with the guarded scalpel. After the incision is made, it is essential that the skin is kept still and taut else the track into the airway can be lost. The person performing the cricothyroidotomy will only have one hand free to insert the tube. An introducer is inserted through the incision and the tube passed up to its flange. The introducer is then removed and the catheter mount connected. The device can then be connected to a ventilation device and the person ventilated. The position of the tube should be checked and then the tube should be anchored in place using the ties provided.

Drugs used in treating airway problems

While up to this point the chapter has largely dealt with airway problems that affect the upper airway, it is important not to forget that airway problems can result from a problem in the lower airway. Asthma is probably the best example of this. In asthma, an inflammatory response occurs in the lower airways, narrowing some of the airways causing a reversible obstruction to airflow. Drug therapy can be used to correct this inflammation, although additional supportive therapies may be needed until these agents can take effect. The aim of the drug treatments is to dilate the airway and if this proves insufficient alone to resolve the problem, then steroid medicines can be given to suppress the inflammation.

Beta-2 agonists such as salbutamol are given to encourage the smooth muscle in the airways to dilate. If this is not effective alone, then an anticholinergic drug can be added such as ipratropium. Anticholinergic drugs encourage muscles to relax by removing the natural stimulus they have to be slightly constricted at all times. This results in dilation of the airway by a different mechanism. Finally, steroids such as hydrocortisone or prednisolone can be given if the preceding steps are failing to provide adequate resolution. More detailed information on the management of asthma can be found in the British Thoracic Society guidelines for the management of asthma (see Further reading).

Airway summary

While a range of methods and devices can be used to secure the airway, what is singly most important is that an airway is opened and secured. In truth, it matters little which technique is used; what is most important is that a free flow of air through the airway can be achieved and maintained while exposing the patient to the least risk possible.

Recognising and resolving breathing problems

Once the airway has been secured, the next stage is to assess and support a person's breathing. In Chapter 3, a process for screening for acute illness was described and this included searching for signs of breathing problems. In this chapter you are encouraged to become more deductive and start to consider what the possible cause or causes of the breathing problem may be. The common management strategies used to resolve breathing problems will also be explained.

Resolving breathing problems in the short term is relatively simple, though the definitive care which follows can be more complex. Correcting breathing problems centres on the optimisation of ventilation and oxygenation. Achieving this is a stepped approach that can be escalated according to the patient's need. Strategies that are employed in optimising breathing include:

- Ensuring that the chest and lungs can expand fully
- Adding oxygen to the air the patient breathes
- Recruiting more functional lung.

Chest expansion

Expansion of the chest and with it the lungs is the principal action that brings about ventilation of the lungs. For expansion to occur, not only must the chest wall be intact, but neuromuscular function must be preserved. If one of these fails, then chest expansion will become abnormal, leading to a ventilation problem. The expansion of the chest can be tested by simple palpation. There are two types of expansion that should be assessed: anterior–posterior (AP) expansion and outward expansion. To assess AP expansion, place both hands with the palms facing downwards on the upper chest. Then wait for the person to take a breath. If possible, ask the person to take a deep breath. Normal expansion is indicated by symmetrical movement on each side of the chest.

The assessment of outward expansion is slightly more tricky to perform. The lower portion of the lateral chest is grasped with the fingers open and the thumbs off the chest during exhalation. With the skin held on the chest bring the thumbs together in the centre of the chest. Then ask the person to take a deep breath. You should see the thumbs move outwards and turn inwards. Again normal movement is indicated by symmetrical movement. Abnormal expansion is indicated by a thumb that does not move, indicating reduced expansion. Thumbs that move outwards, but not inwards, indicates hyperinflation of the chest, a feature of COPD, among others things.

For some of the failures of chest expansion there is little that can be done other than to ventilate the person artificially. This will be the case when there are severe rib fractures causing a flail segment, or if the nervous innervation has been damaged. The interventions that can restore chest expansion involve situations in which there is separation of the pleural layers. Air, blood, fluid and pus can enter the pleural space reducing the lungs' ability to expand. The medically correct names for these conditions are air pneumothorax, blood haemothorax, fluid pleural effusions and pus empyema, respectively. The treatment for these conditions is to remove the matter causing the problem.

Tension pneumothorax is a special type of pneumothorax that requires rapid identification and immediate management if haemodynamic collapse is to be averted. In tension pneumothorax, air progressively enters the pleural space and the pressure inside the pleura increases. This high pressure in the pleura eventually displaces other vital structures in the chest and can obstruct blood flow in the chest. In spontaneously breathing individuals this condition can develop steadily. In those who are ventilated, this condition can develop rapidly. Eventually, if not recognised and treated, tension pneumothorax can result in cardiac arrest. Tension pneumothorax can be difficult to detect, although it should be suspected in patients with chest injuries, those who have been ventilated or have an underlying lung pathology and who suddenly deteriorate with increasing difficulty in breathing, hypoxia, reduced chest expansion and distension of the neck veins.

The management of a tension pneumothorax is to relieve the pressure of air that has formed within the pleural space. This is achieved by inserting a needle through the chest wall into the pleural space so that the air can drain into the atmosphere. The correct name for this procedure is needle thoracentesis, also sometimes referred to as a needle decompression. This procedure is normally performed by medical staff, although others such as paramedics and suitably trained nurses may also undertake the procedure.

During the procedure, a large-bore (14-gauge) intravenous cannula is inserted into the second intercostal space in the mid-clavicular line, immediately above the bone. This position is chosen so to avoid damaging the neurovascular bundle that is present on the base of each rib. Once the cannula is inserted, the needle is withdrawn and successful decompression is indicated by a sudden hiss of air from the cannula and a subsequent improvement in the patient's condition. The cannula is left in place until a chest drain can be sited. Occasionally, particularly in obese patients, it may not be possible to decompress the chest in the second intercostal space and the lateral chest wall is penetrated instead. As well as treating pneumothorax, needle thoracentesis can also cause pneumothorax in a proportion of patients in which the condition is not already present, so an emergency chest X-ray should be performed to confirm the diagnosis in spontaneously breathing patients if the clinical circumstances allow.

Restriction to chest expansion can occur when the skin on the chest wall is burned. Inflammation in the burned tissue tightens the skin covering the chest wall and prevents it from expanding fully. Escharotomy is a surgical procedure that involves cutting into the skin of the chest sequentially. This relieves the constriction and allows the chest to expand. This treatment is radical and often palliative.

Adding oxygen to the breathed air

Oxygen therapy is a long-established treatment for hypoxaemia, and oxygen has become one of the most commonly used drugs in hospital. The use of oxygen in the past has been erratic and without a true evidence base. This has led to suboptimal care, exposing patients to the risks associated with uncorrected hypoxia and oxygen overdose. The British Thoracic Society (BTS) has recently published guidelines (O'Driscoll et al., 2008) on the use of emergency oxygen and hopefully, when deployed in practice, these guidelines will serve to standardise practice in this area. The main focus of the BTS guideline is to assert that oxygen therapy should be goal directed and only given where there is a demonstrated reason to do so. This means that oxygen should be given only when the patient is demonstrated to be hypoxic and that oxygen should not be given routinely to treat breathlessness. In addition to this guideline, the BTS also recommends that high-concentration oxygen is given via a non-rebreathe mask to all patients who have the conditions listed in Box 4.9. The non-rebreathe mask (Figure 4.10, A) allows for the administration of the highest concentration of oxygen out of all the oxygen delivery devices used in spontaneously breathing individuals. It has an integral oxygen reservoir which must be filled with oxygen before it is placed on the patient's face. A series of valves in the mask helps to reduce inhalation of ambient room air. The exact concentration of oxygen that is delivered by this type is variable and dependent on a number of factors, although it is likely to be in the region of 80%.

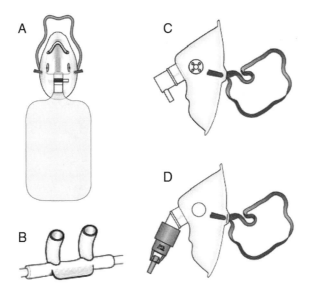

FIGURE 4.10   *Oxygen delivery devices. A, non-rebreathe mask; B, nasal cannula; C, simple oxygen mask; D, Venturi mask.*
Images reproduced with the kind permission of Intersurgical.

BOX 4.9   *Conditions to be treated with high-concentration oxygen therapy via a non-rebreathe mask*

- Post cardiac/respiratory arrest
- Shock
- Sepsis
- Major trauma
- Near-drowning
- Anaphylaxis
- Major pulmonary haemorrhage
- Major head injury
- Carbon monoxide poisoning
- Status epilepticus
- Previously healthy people with a SaO_2% of 85% or less

(Source: O'Driscoll et al., 2008)

If oxygen is to be given to correct hypoxaemia, it is necessary to establish how much oxygen is in the blood. This is achieved using a pulse oximeter. The results from the pulse oximeter are expressed as the patient's SaO_2%. The SaO_2% provides an estimation of the amount of oxygen that is bound to haemoglobin in the blood. The BTS (O'Driscoll et al., 2008)

recommends that oxygen should be administered to achieve a target SaO_2%
of 94–98% for most acutely ill patients or 88–92% for those at risk of type 2
respiratory failure. Patients at risk of type 2 respiratory failure include those
with COPD or other chronic chest conditions such as cystic fibrosis.

Successful titration of an oxygen dose requires that:

- The patient's SaO_2% is monitored
  - At baseline
  - In response to oxygen therapy
- The correct oxygen delivery device is used
- The correct flow of oxygen is administered through the delivery device
- Records are made of:
  - The patient's SaO_2%
  - The delivery device in use if any
  - The oxygen flow given if any
- Changes are made to both increase and decrease oxygen dose when indicated.

The person's SaO_2% should be assessed each time their vital signs are
recorded. This should be interpreted in the light of whether the person is
breathing room air or supplemental oxygen. An SaO_2% of 93% or less in a
previously healthy individual indicates the presence of hypoxaemia. Where
this is seen in a person not currently receiving oxygen therapy it is an
indication to start such treatment. If the person is receiving oxygen therapy
the oxygen dose should be increased to achieve the target saturation. Being
able to titrate the oxygen dose correctly requires an understanding of oxygen flow, how different delivery devices handle oxygen, and the fraction
of inspired oxygen that is eventually administered to the patient via the
delivery device.

Oxygen is dispensed from the wall supply or cylinder in litres per
minute (LPM). Anecdotal observations suggest that many health professionals consider that this value is the dose of oxygen that is given to the
person. This is a misconception as the dose of oxygen that is given to the
patient will depend not only on the flow of oxygen, but also on the delivery device that the oxygen is put through. This is illustrated by the fact that
if the same flow of oxygen is put through different delivery devices, a different dose of oxygen will be administered to the patient. More correctly,
the oxygen dose should be considered as the percentage of oxygen that the
person breathes in from the delivery device. This percentage is referred to
as the fraction of inspired oxygen (FiO_2%). Room air contains 21% oxygen
so the FiO_2% of room air is 21%. The aim of giving oxygen therapy is to
increase the FiO_2% above this level.

Probably the most important thing to note about oxygen masks is that they are not all the same and each type has specific qualities and indications. As a result of this, oxygen delivery devices are not interchangeable and diligence in choosing and using an oxygen delivery device is required. Oxygen delivery devices can be classified as:

- Fixed performance
- Variable performance.

Fixed performance devices deliver a fixed concentration of oxygen to the patient, whereas variable performance devices deliver a variable dose of oxygen to the patient depending on both the rate and depth of the patient's breathing as well as the oxygen flow. Box 4.10 shows how different devices are classified and images of the different devices are shown in Figure 4.10.

BOX 4.10   Classification of oxygen delivery devices

- Fixed performance devices:

  o Venturi mask

- Variable performance devices:

  o Nasal cannula
  o Simple oxygen mask
  o High concentration (non-rebreathe mask)
  o Bag valve mask resuscitator with oxygen reservoir
  o Tracheotomy mask.

The fixed performance devices, essentially the Venturi masks, deliver a fixed FiO_2%. The exact amount of oxygen that is given to the patient is governed by the colour-coded tip that is attached to the mask, the flow of oxygen into the mask and the exact constituents of room air. Concentrations of 24–50% oxygen can be given using this type of mask. Other devices such as the simple oxygen mask, the non-rebreathe mask and nasal cannula do not produce a fixed FiO_2% and the dose of oxygen given to the patient will depend on the:

- Flow of oxygen into the device
- Person's respiratory rate
- Depth of breathing
- Amount of air that is also breathed in (air entrapment).

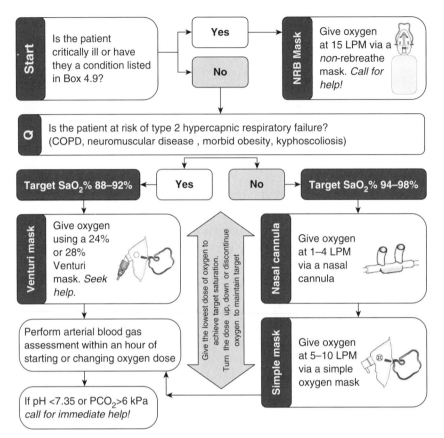

FIGURE 4.11   *Protocol for the initial titration of oxygen therapy in spontaneously breathing adults. LPM, litres per minute; COPD, chronic obstructive pulmonary disease.*

Due to the unpredictable nature at which these variable devices perform they are less suitable for use where controlled amounts of oxygen need to be given to a patient. The BTS (O'Driscoll et al., 2008) recommends that most stable patients can be safely given oxygen using a nasal cannula for flow rates of up to 4 LPM or a simple oxygen mask for flow rates of 5 LPM or more. A simple oxygen mask should never be used with flow rates of less than 5 LPM as there is a risk of promoting carbon dioxide retention. Patients at risk of type 2 respiratory failure should initially be given oxygen using either a 24% or 28% Venturi mask until a full assessment of their condition can be made. Figure 4.11 summarises the protocol for the administration of oxygen to a patient.

Recruit more functional lung

The final strategy that can be used to improve oxygenation of the blood is to involve more functional lung tissue in breathing. In real terms increasing

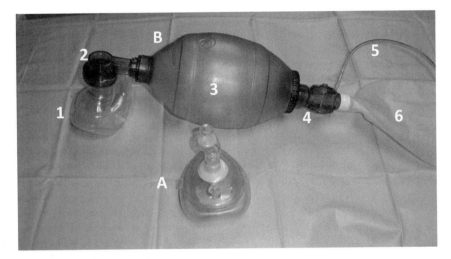

FIGURE 4.12   *Ventilation devices used for intermittent positive pressure ventilation.*
A, pocket mask; B, self-inflating bag; 1, face mask; 2, patient valve, 3; self-inflating bag;
4, inlet valve; 5, oxygen drive line; 6, oxygen reservoir.

the amount of lung that is involved in breathing means increasing the tidal volume – the amount of air moved with each breath. Some strategies also involve maintaining a pressure within the airway at the end of expiration in an effort to keep the air spaces open. This allows maximum time for gas exchange and reduces trauma to the endothelial lining of the airways. The methods that can be used to ventilate the lungs include intermittent positive pressure ventilation and non-invasive ventilation.

Intermittent positive pressure ventilation (IPPV)
IPPV, as the name suggests, involves the application of positive pressure to the lungs intermittently. It is the simplest form of ventilation and its use is of great value in the acutely ill mainly as it can be implemented quickly and simply when the need arises. Mouth-to-mouth resuscitation is a form of positive pressure ventilation, though in the clinical setting mouth-to-mouth resuscitation has lost favour and the wide availability of other ventilation devices makes its use in the main unnecessary. You should consider IPPV in patients who are breathing very rapidly or very slowly. Patients who are not breathing deeply enough to move sufficient air into the lungs will also benefit from IPPV. IPPV is essential if the person has stopped breathing.

One of the easiest of these devices to use is the pocket mask (Figure 4.12, A). This is a device that can be used by a single operator to ventilate the lungs when a person is not breathing normally or not breathing at all. To operate this device it must be first assembled. The one-way valve must be attached to the mask and the mask must be unfolded. If an oxygen inlet is available then oxygen should be connected and set to a flow rate of 8 LPM. If the device does not have an oxygen inlet then oxygen tubing can be placed under the cuff of the mask and a seal made around this. Pocket masks are easier to use when you are standing behind the patient's head rather than at their side. The assembled mask is positioned on the chin and then lowered into position. The seal is then formed by clamping the mask onto the patient's face by placing the thumbs along the upper edge of the mask and applying counter pressure, placing the fingers under the angle of the jaw. The rescuer can then blow air through the mask to inflate the patient's lungs. As air is blown into the mask, the rescuer should check that air is not leaking and that the chest rises.

When ventilating a person artificially without intubation there is a risk that gas can enter the stomach and promote regurgitation of stomach contents, which will further complicate airway management. To reduce this risk it is important to pay attention to the patency of the airway. Optimal head tilt-chin lift should be performed before attempting ventilation in all patients unless it is contraindicated. Breaths should be given slowly over about one second, delivering sufficient air to make the chest rise. Excessive chest rise is not required and increases the risk of regurgitation.

The self-inflating bag (Figure 4.12, B), also known as a bag valve mask device or Ambu bag, is another device that can be used to provide IPPV. The main benefit of the self-inflating bag is that it can provide a higher concentration of oxygen, particularly when used with an oxygen reservoir and flow rates of 10 LPM. However, there are drawbacks to the use of a self-inflating bag, the main ones being that it is difficult for one person to operate when connected to a mask, and its overzealous use can cause gastric inflation. To overcome these problems either a two-rescuer technique is used, one holding the mask in place and maintaining a clear airway, with a second rescuer squeezing the bag; alternatively, an intermediate airway device can be inserted and ventilation provided via this device by a single rescuer. This second option also reduces the risk of gastric inflation and offers greater airway protection.

To operate a self-inflating bag it should be assembled according to the manufacturer's instructions. If a mask is being used it should be attached to the patient valve. The person holding the mask on the patient's face should be positioned at the patient's head. The person squeezing the bag should be at the patient's side. The mask is held in position as described earlier for the pocket mask. The bag is then compressed between the hands of the second rescuer for one second. Chest rise should be seen when the bag is compressed. If any air leak is detected the person holding the mask should reposition it to eliminate this.

If an intermediate airway device can be inserted without delay and the patient is sufficiently unconscious to tolerate the insertion of such a device, then this is the preferred method of using the self-inflating bag. This method requires only one rescuer, freeing up the second person for other tasks. In addition, airway care is of a better standard with less risk of pulmonary aspiration of gastric contents and, finally, should chest compressions be necessary then this can be performed continuously without pause for ventilations. When using a self-inflating bag with an intermediate airway device it should be connected to the device using a catheter mount. The rescuer should then squeeze the bag with both hands.

Mechanical ventilators are devices that provide a more permanent solution for ventilation than either of the above-described two methods. Ventilators are complex devices that offer many different ways in which they can support breathing. Specialist training is needed to operate a ventilator safely and their use is not common outside the critical care area.

Non-invasive ventilation (NIV)

Traditional formal mechanical ventilation requires intubation or tracheotomy and, because of this, ventilation was deemed invasive and required admission to the intensive care unit. Recent technological developments have realised the opportunity to continuously ventilate a person without the need for intubation or tracheotomy. This type of ventilation uses a face mask, making it a popular alternative to invasive ventilation for suitable patients. There are essentially two types of NIV in use:

- Continuous positive airway pressure (CPAP)
- Bi-level positive airway pressure (BiPAP).

The main indication for CPAP is in the treatment of obstructive sleep apnoea (OSA). In OSA flaccid tissue obstructs the airway during sleep, leading to periods of apnoea. This gives rise to a ventilation problem which increases the carbon dioxide content of the blood, raises blood pressure and reduces the person's sleep quality. CPAP maintains a minimum pressure within the airways and this pressure splints the tissues, preventing the obstruction and allowing ventilation to take place unimpeded.

BiPAP builds on the technology used in CPAP. In BiPAP, as the name suggests, two pressure levels are set, an inspiratory pressure and an expiratory pressure. During inspiration the patient's breath is assisted by pressurised air being forced into the lungs. On expiration the minimum expiratory pressure prevents the flaccid airways from collapsing and improves ventilation. In type 2 respiratory failure this should facilitate the removal of carbon dioxide from the blood. In cardiogenic pulmonary oedema the constant positive pressure in the lungs drives the fluid in the lungs back into the circulation.

BiPAP has established a role in the management of acute type 2 respiratory failure secondary to COPD, which is not responsive to maximal medical therapies such as bronchodilators, steroids and oxygen. BiPAP is also used in the treatment of cardiogenic pulmonary oedema. The Royal College of Physicians has published a guideline on the use of BiPAP in patients with COPD and type 2 respiratory failure (Royal College of Physicians (RCP), 2008). In this guideline, details are provided regarding who is suitable and who is not suitable for treatment with NIV. Details of how NIV should be provided and the service context in which NIV is provided are also included. The RCP (2008) recommends that NIV is indicated in the management of patients with:

- COPD
- Chest wall deformity, neuromuscular disorder, decompensated OSA
- Cardiogenic pulmonary oedema, unresponsive to CPAP

where there is respiratory acidosis (PaCO$_2$ >6.0 kPa, pH <7.35 or H$^+$ >45 nmol/L), which persists despite maximal medical treatment and appropriate controlled oxygen therapy. The RCP also acknowledges that patients with pH <7.25 or H$^+$ >56 nmol/L respond less well and should be managed in a high-dependency or intensive care unit rather than a respiratory ward. The RCP (2008) recommends that the clinical state of the patient should be:

- Sick but not moribund
- Able to protect their airway
- Conscious and cooperative
- Haemodynamically stable.

There should also be no excessive respiratory secretions and few co-morbidities.

NIV is mainly contraindicated in patients (RCP, 2008) with:

- Facial burns/trauma/recent facial or upper airway surgery
- Vomiting
- Fixed upper airway obstruction
- Undrained pneumothorax.

NIV is delivered initially using a tight-fitting full face mask. This can trigger anxiety in patients and psychological support is required to assist patients to overcome this and comply with the treatment. Patients being treated with NIV need close observation and will require regular assessment of arterial blood gas tensions. NIV should be delivered only by staff who have been specifically trained to do so.

Problems with ventilation

Ventilation of the lungs by whichever strategy reverses normal physiology. In place of a negative pressure being created within the chest by movement of the diaphragm and the chest wall, inspiration is forced by positive pressure air being driven into the lungs. While resolving in part the ventilation/oxygenation problem this reverse in physiology can cause a number of other problems for the patient.

The negative pressure that causes air to be drawn into the lungs during normal breathing also assists venous return to the heart. Positive pressure ventilation conversely reduces venous return. In turn this reduces cardiac output and can worsen haemodynamic stability. The lungs can be damaged directly by positive pressure ventilation in a process called barotrauma. If excessively high pressures are used to ventilate the lungs or the lungs are weakened, there is a possibility that part of the lung can rupture, causing a pneumothorax. If ventilation continues then this simple pneumothorax can quickly become a tension pneumothorax. A patient who is being ventilated and experiences sudden deterioration should be investigated for the possibility of pneumothorax.

Conclusion

Oxygen is an essential component for cell energy production. The purpose of the respiratory system is to oxygenate the blood so that the circulatory system can transport oxygen to the cells of the body, where it is used to produce maximal amounts of energy. Carbon dioxide is a byproduct of cell energy production. When dissolved in blood, carbon dioxide makes the blood more acidic. The respiratory system has a role in regulating the acidity of the blood by blowing off carbon dioxide. Where a problem develops with the body's ability either to take in oxygen or rid itself of carbon dioxide, respiratory failure is said to occur.

Problems with the airway and breathing occur frequently in those who are acutely ill. Consistent with other aspects of acute illness management, all too often these problems go unnoticed and fail to receive appropriate management. This worsens patient outcomes and contributes to increased mortality among those who become acutely ill while in hospital.

Problems can develop with respiratory function for a number of reasons. Compromise or occlusion of the airway acutely impairs breathing and can lead directly to respiratory failure. Alternatively a problem with the lungs themselves can occur and result in a type of respiratory failure which may present acutely or chronically.

Management of the patient with impending or established respiratory failure involves recognising that the person is in distress and taking action to correct this. The earlier that intervention is provided, the more successful it is likely to be and the less invasive techniques are likely to be sufficient. If basic techniques fail to correct the situation rapidly, the patient's care should be escalated to ensure they receive more advanced methods of support immediately.

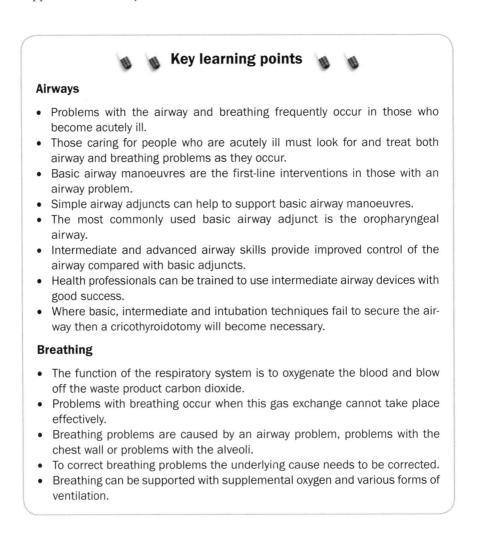

Key learning points

Airways

- Problems with the airway and breathing frequently occur in those who become acutely ill.
- Those caring for people who are acutely ill must look for and treat both airway and breathing problems as they occur.
- Basic airway manoeuvres are the first-line interventions in those with an airway problem.
- Simple airway adjuncts can help to support basic airway manoeuvres.
- The most commonly used basic airway adjunct is the oropharyngeal airway.
- Intermediate and advanced airway skills provide improved control of the airway compared with basic adjuncts.
- Health professionals can be trained to use intermediate airway devices with good success.
- Where basic, intermediate and intubation techniques fail to secure the airway then a cricothyroidotomy will become necessary.

Breathing

- The function of the respiratory system is to oxygenate the blood and blow off the waste product carbon dioxide.
- Problems with breathing occur when this gas exchange cannot take place effectively.
- Breathing problems are caused by an airway problem, problems with the chest wall or problems with the alveoli.
- To correct breathing problems the underlying cause needs to be corrected.
- Breathing can be supported with supplemental oxygen and various forms of ventilation.

🔋 🔋 Self-assessment questions 🔋 🔋

1   Which of the following could cause a ventilation problem in the lungs?

   A   Anaemia
   B   Chronic obstructive pulmonary disease
   C   Hypoxaemia
   D   Respiratory failure
   E   All of the above

2   Hypercapnic respiratory failure is most likely to occur in those patients who have:

   A   Oxygenation problems
   B   Ventilation problems
   C   Breathing problems
   D   Hypovolaemia
   E   Histotoxic hypoxia

3   An SaO_2% equal to or less than .... in an otherwise healthy person indicates that hypoxaemia is present.

   A   85%
   B   90%
   C   92%
   D   93%
   E   98%

4   Which one of the following is a sign of an upper airway obstruction?

   A   Chest pain
   B   Low blood pressure
   C   Unequal chest expansion
   D   Vomiting
   E   Snoring sounds

5   To identify the correct size for an oropharyngeal airway you should measure it:

   A   Against the person's ring finger
   B   From the tip of the nose to the angle of the ear lobe
   C   From the incisors to the angle of the jaw
   D   From the chin to the top of the ear
   E   From the chin to the hyoid

6   In type 2 respiratory failure a person will have:

   A   Low levels of oxygen in the blood only
   B   Low levels of oxygen and low levels of carbon dioxide in the blood
   C   High levels of carbon dioxide in the blood

(Continued)

(Continued)

    D   An SaO_2% of less than 93%
    E   A $PaCO_2$ of 3 kPa

7   Chest expansion will be reduced in which one of the following conditions?

    A   Tension pneumothorax
    B   Pulmonary oedema
    C   Metabolic acidosis
    D   Pulmonary embolism
    E   Cor pulmonale

8   The best device to give oxygen to a stable patient without COPD is:

    A   Non-rebreathe mask
    B   Venturi mask
    C   Simple oxygen mask
    D   Nasal cannula
    E   Bag valve mask

9   People with which one of the following diagnoses should receive oxygen via a non-rebreathe mask?

    A   Myocardial infarction
    B   Cerebrovascular accident
    C   Hypertension
    D   Anaphylaxis
    E   All of the above

10   Non-invasive ventilation is a useful treatment for which one of the following conditions?

    A   Acute hypercapnic respiratory failure
    B   Acute hypoxaemic respiratory failure
    C   Acute pneumonia
    D   Pulmonary embolism
    E   All types of respiratory failure

Answers

1B, 2B, 3D, 4E, 5C, 6C, 7A, 8D, 9D, 10A.

Further reading

Bourke, S.J. (2007) *Lecture Notes on Respiratory Medicine*. Oxford: Blackwell Publishing. This text expands on the content of this chapter by providing more detail about how lung dysfunction can occur and how to assess and treat respiratory pathologies.

Clancy, J. and McVicar, A. (2009) *Physiology and Anatomy for Nurses and Healthcare Practitioners: A Homeostatic Approach*. London: Hodder Arnold.
This is a well-respected text that will enable you to deepen your knowledge about the anatomy and physiology that surrounds respiratory function.

British Thoracic Society and Scottish Intercollegiate Guideline Networks (2008) *British Guideline on the Management of Asthma; A National Clinical Guideline*. London: BTS. Available online at www.brit-thoracic.org.uk.
This is an important guideline that describes best practice in the assessment and management of patients with asthma. Other guidelines that relate to the care of those with breathing problems are available on the BTS website.

O'Driscoll, B., Howard, L. and Davison, A. on behalf of the British Thoracic Society Emergency Oxygen Guideline Development Group, a subgroup of the British Thoracic Society Standards of Care Committee (2008) 'Guideline for emergency oxygen use in adult patients', *Thorax*, 63 (Supplement VI).
This guideline provides important direction for healthcare staff in how to administer oxygen to those who are acutely ill.

5

Understanding and resolving problems with the circulation

Chapter aims

By the end of this chapter you should be able to:

- Explain how problems with circulation develop
- Take action to resolve problems with circulation

The circulation of blood provides an important transport system for the body. At times of acute illness the circulation can fail for a number of reasons causing a condition known as shock. Shock has been defined by Eaton (1999) as 'a condition characterised by impaired cellular function as a result of a reduction in the effective circulating blood volume, resulting in an inadequate supply of oxygen and nutrients to the cells, tissues and organs, inadequate oxygen utilisation and inadequate removal of waste products'. Shock therefore represents a life-threatening condition with the potential to seriously upset homeostasis, causing cellular dysfunction, injury and death.

In Chapter 2, some of the changes that can lead to shock were explained and in Chapter 3 a system for recognising the shocked patient was outlined. In this chapter the different types of shock will be described

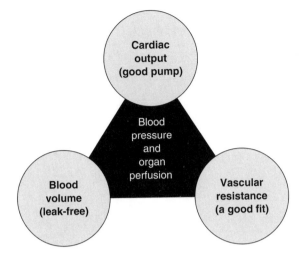

FIGURE 5.1   *The perfusion triad.*

in detail and the treatment required to resolve these conditions will be explained.

The perfusion triad

All the tissues of the body need to have blood coursing through them if they are to be well nourished and their waste products removed. This flow of blood is called perfusion. To understand perfusion, it is helpful to think of the perfusion triad (Figure 5.1). The perfusion triad explains in simple terms the required components of organ perfusion. It recognises that for a person to have normal perfusion they must have a functioning heart to pump the blood, and they must have healthy blood to pump and healthy blood vessels ('pipes') to circulate the blood around the body, eventually returning it to the heart. If one of these essential components fails, then circulation will be impaired and shock will develop. When the effectiveness of perfusion is questioned, it is helpful to think: is this a pump problem, a blood volume problem, a pipes problem or a combination of these? This can help to identify the cause of the perfusion failure and guide management.

Shock can be brought about in a number of different ways. The different types of shock are listed in Box 5.1 under the headings of the perfusion triad. The remainder of this chapter will explain the perfusion triad, the types of shock that occur and the initial treatment that is required.

BOX 5.1   Classifications of shock

Blood volume failure

- Hypovolaemic

Cardiac pump failure

- Cardiogenic

Vascular resistance (pipe) failure

- Obstructive
- Distributive

  - Anaphylactic
  - Septic
  - Neurogenic

A good cardiac output (a good pump)

Let us start by considering the role of the heart in pumping blood. In order for the heart to pump effectively it must be healthy. In short this requires that:

- The muscle of the heart is functional
- The conduction system in the heart is undamaged and in control
- The valves in the heart are functional
- The sac surrounding the heart is free from excessive fluid and not unduly tight.

When any one of these points fail, the heart pump becomes less effective and shock can develop. Shock caused by pump failure is termed cardiogenic shock.

Damage to the muscle of the heart

The most common cause of damage to the heart muscle is coronary artery disease (CAD). In CAD, the coronary arteries that supply the heart muscle become damaged by plaques in their walls (Figure 5.2). As these plaques develop, they impair the blood supply to the heart muscle, which reduces the amount of energy that the heart has. While at rest this may not cause the affected person any major problems, when they exert themselves or become emotionally distressed the heart rate increases and with it the amount of energy the heart requires. You will recall that energy is manufactured from oxygen and glucose supplied by

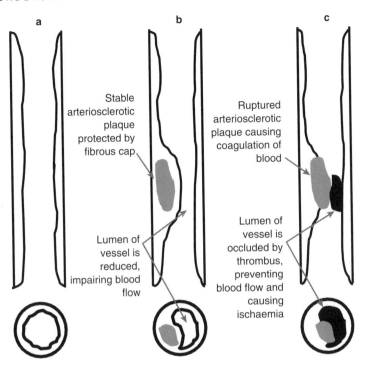

FIGURE 5.2   *Coronary artery plaques obstructing blood flow. (a) Normal vessel,*
(b) small stable plaque and (c) plaque rupture and thrombus formation leading to
vessel occlusion.

the blood. It follows that, if the blood supply available to the heart is impaired by narrowing of the coronary arteries, when there is demand for additional blood, the supply cannot be maintained at the rate required. The heart becomes energy-deficient. Clinically this causes some chest pain. If the chest pain resolves quickly and completely with rest or treatment with glyceryl trinitrate (GTN), this condition is termed stable angina.

Occasionally, plaques in the coronary artery can rupture, resulting in a blood clot forming within the coronary artery, which in turn obstructs blood flow to the heart muscle (Figure 5.2c). When this occurs, myocardial infarction is the diagnosis and rapid medical intervention is required to restore blood flow, or the portion of the heart muscle supplied by that coronary artery can die if no adequate collateral blood supply is in place. In physiological terms, heart muscle that has no blood supply has no available energy. This means that the infarcted portion of the heart is unable to contract. The size and location of the infarct will determine how serious its impact is on the patient. Infarcts that compromise a large proportion of the left ventricular wall can seriously reduce cardiac output and cause severe pulmonary oedema.

Early recognition and optimal management of patients with myocardial infarction reduces mortality and morbidity both in the short and long terms. When chest pain or discomfort which may radiate to the arms, abdomen, neck, jaw and back is present along with other cardiac symptoms such as those listed in Box 5.2, the patient may be having a myocardial infarction and warrants further immediate investigation.

BOX 5.2 Symptoms suggestive of an acute coronary syndrome

- Chest pain that may radiate into the arms, back, abdomen, neck or jaw
- Shortness of breath (dyspnoea)
- Nausea
- Vomiting
- Sweating

N.B.: Patients with diabetes who are older or who are female, can display atypical presentation. This can include the silent myocardial infarction phenomenon, where this condition occurs without causing chest pain.

At the point of patient presentation it can be difficult to differentiate between those patients who have angina and those who have an established myocardial infarction. Not all myocardial infarctions are the same and it can take time for one to manifest. For these reasons, among others, patients who present with cardiac symptoms should be considered as having an acute coronary syndrome (ACS) until it can be proven that they do not have it or their symptoms are better explained by another diagnosis. ACS is an umbrella term that encompasses the conditions of:

- ST elevation myocardial infarction (STEMI)
- Non-ST elevation myocardial infarction (NSTEMI)
- Unstable angina pectoris (UAP).

To determine the difference between a STEMI and a NSTEMI, a 12-lead electrocardiograph (ECG) is required. The ECG produces an electrical picture of the heart looking from 12 different vantage points. Part of the ECG, the ST segment (Figure 5.3a) is particularly sensitive to changes caused by ischaemic damage to the heart muscle. In health the ST segment

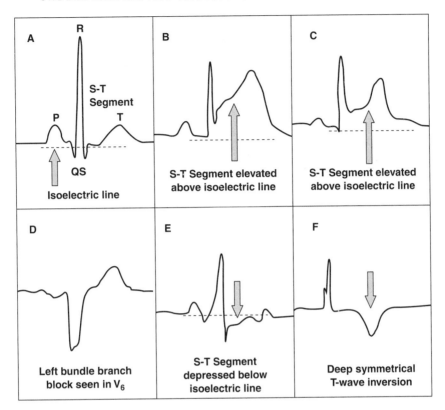

FIGURE 5.3   *ST changes. (a) Normal ST segment, (b) ST elevation in the limb leads, (c) ST segment elevation in the praecordial leads, (d) left bundle branch block pattern in V₆, (e) non-specific ST segment depressions and (f) deep symmetrical T-wave inversions.*

is level with the isoelectric line. The ST segment can deviate from this line and when this happens a pathology is present.

The most important change is that of ST segment elevation. ST elevation is defined as a movement of the ST segment above the isoelectric line by one small square in two or more adjacent limb leads (I, II, III, aV_R, aV_L, aV_F) and/or two small squares in two or more adjacent praecordial leads ($V_1, V_2, V_3, V_4, V_5, V_6$). These changes are illustrated in Figure 5.3b and 5.3c. Where the ECG shows ST elevation satisfying the above criteria, a STEMI is said to have occurred. Another ECG finding that indicates the presence of STEMI is the development of presumably new left bundle branch block on the ECG. This occurs when ischaemic damage to the heart blocks the passage of electrical signals down the left bundle branch, producing a broad ECG complex. An example of how this typically appears is shown in Figure 5.3d, which displays the complex viewed from lead V_6.

While the ECG is important in making the diagnosis of STEMI, it is of lesser value in diagnosing NSTEMI and UAP. In both of these conditions, the ECG can be totally normal despite severe coronary artery lesions being present. Alternatively, the ECG shows non-specific signs of ischaemia such as ST segment depressions (Figures 5.3e) or deep symmetrical T-wave inversions (Figure 5.3f). These findings are non-specific and not in themselves diagnostic of NSTEMI or UAP. To differentiate between NSTEMI and UAP a further test is needed. In NSTEMI some cardiac muscle dies. In UAP the muscle suffers ischaemic challenge, but this challenge is not sufficient to bring about death of cardiac muscle cells. When cardiac muscle cells die, they release certain chemical markers. The most important of these are troponin T and troponin I. A blood test for troponins can be made and this is a useful discriminator between NSTEMI and UAP. It takes time for these markers to be released and so one drawback of the test is that it can only be performed 12 hours after the onset of symptoms if the result is to be conclusive. A positive test for troponins supports the diagnosis of NSTEMI and a negative test suggests UAP as the diagnosis.

Treatment for acute coronary syndrome

The definitive management of STEMI, NSTEMI and UAP differs slightly, although the supportive therapies used in the management of ACS are common to each of the conditions. In STEMI, emergency revascularisation is the ultimate aim and helps to reduce morbidity and mortality in both the long and short term by limiting the ischaemic time and preserving heart muscle. In NSTEMI and UAP, as the diagnosis cannot be made immediately, primary revascularisation is not possible. During the early stages of ACS, common supportive care can be given to limit the impact of the ischaemia, no matter what the ultimate diagnosis turns out to be. These early treatments consist of:

- Analgesia:
  - GTN
  - Morphine
- Antiplatelet therapy:
  - aspirin
- Oxygen when hypoxia is present ($SaO_2\% \leq 93\%$).

Cardiac ischaemia, no matter what its cause, is commonly associated with severe pain. Relieving pain is not only important for patient comfort but the analgesic strategies used in ACS also invoke useful physiological changes that help to improve cardiac function. Initial efforts for relieving pain in patients with ACS should centre on the use of GTN. GTN is a nitrate-based drug that brings about dilation of blood vessels. The aim of giving nitrates is to dilate the collateral arteries, increasing the delivery of blood to the areas of the heart that have become ischaemic, thus mitigating the ischaemia (Rang et al., 2007). Nitrates exercise a systemic effect on the body, which also helps to relieve ischaemia in the heart by reducing the cardiac workload (Rang et al., 2007). Dilating blood vessels has the effect of lowering blood pressure and GTN should only be given if the patient's blood pressure is above 90 mmHg systolic. GTN is available in a variety of presentations. The most convenient for use in the initial stages of ACS is a metered dose pump spray that delivers 400 micrograms of GTN per spray. The spray is directed under the patient's tongue and it is absorbed through the mucosal membrane. The dose can be repeated if pain persists up to a total of 1.2 mg (three sprays) provided that the patient's blood pressure remains above 90 mmHg. A benefit of GTN is that it can be administered quickly and simply while intravenous access is being obtained.

Where pain fails to respond to GTN, morphine is the drug of choice. Morphine should be given intravenously and titrated against the patient's response. The initial starting dose is 3–5 mg, repeated until the patient is pain-free or the maximal safe dose is reached.

When plaque ruptures in the coronary artery, a chain reaction takes place that results in a blood clot being formed. The changes that lead to the development of a clot can be very simply explained in two stages. First, a fibrin scaffolding is formed, and, second, activated platelets attach to this scaffolding and form a clot. Antiplatelet therapy such as aspirin and clopidogrel can be given to prevent the aggregation of platelets in an effort to limit the size of the primary clot and to prevent further clots from forming.

Oxygen is given when there is demonstrated hypoxia (SaO_2% equal to or less than 93%). Where oxygen therapy is indicated it should be titrated as described in Chapter 4. Other treatments such as heparin, angiotensin-converting enzyme inhibitors and beta-blockers also have a role in the management of myocardial infarction, but their use is a little more complicated and beyond the scope of this chapter.

Definitive management of STEMI

The definitive management of STEMI is concerned with reopening the occluded coronary artery. There are essentially two options through which this can be achieved: fibrinolytic therapy and primary percutaneous coronary intervention (PPCI). Fibrinolytic therapy is the older of these two treatments. It involves administering a drug that dissolves the fibrin scaffolding which holds the offending clot together. One of the main problems with fibrinolytic therapy is that it is not specific to blood clots in the coronary arteries and it will dissolve useful clots elsewhere in the body and can cause bleeding that can lead to stroke or death. Fibrinolytic therapy therefore is not suitable for all patients. Also, fibrinolytic therapy is only useful in the first few hours after the onset of symptoms as the fibrin scaffold becomes less soluble after this time and the benefits gained from administering fibrinolytic drugs are reduced.

PPCI involve passing a catheter into the coronary artery with the aid of an X-ray. A balloon on the outside of the catheter is then inflated at the location of the blockage. A stent, which is a kind of intraluminal splint, is also usually inserted at the same time. As PPCI does not involve the administration of drugs to dissolve blood clots, it is not associated with the same risk of bleeding. This makes PPCI suitable for use in a wider range of patients and is now the preferred treatment for most patients with STEMI. PPCI is not without risk; rupture of the coronary artery can occur and for this reason it is normally performed only in centres with facilities to address such a complication should it arise.

Non-ischaemic causes of heart muscle damage

As well as infarction, infections can cause inflammation of the heart muscle and limit its pumping ability. While these are less common than ischaemic causes, it is important not to forget this possibility.

Damage to the conduction system of the heart

The heart muscle is stimulated to contract (beat) by an electrical current. A graphical representation of the electrical activity of the heart can be seen on the ECG. In health, electrical current passes through the heart and creates an organised heart beat. This normal rhythm is called normal sinus rhythm. Illness states can interrupt this normal passage of electricity through the heart, and then an arrhythmia is said to have occurred. The understanding and recognition of both normal and abnormal heart rhythms are the subject of Chapter 6. Here the discussion of arrhythmias intends to illustrate how they can cause shock without getting entrenched in the details over exactly which arrhythmia is to blame.

When arrhythmia occurs, the heart muscle receives an abnormal message stimulating it to beat. The electrical stimulation of the heart muscle tells the heart when and how to beat. Changes from normal electrical conduction means that the heart beats abnormally and this can reduce cardiac output. When an arrhythmia occurs there are three possible outcomes that lead to the development of circulatory failure. These are:

- The heart beats too slowly
- The heart beats too fast
- The heart is not beating in a coordinated way and no cardiac output is produced (cardiac arrest occurs).

Cardiac output is the amount of blood pumped out of the left ventricle in one minute. It is calculated by establishing how much blood is pumped out of the left ventricle in one beat, the stroke volume, and multiplying this by the heart rate. When the heart rate is very slow, the heart is beating too infrequently to maintain cardiac output. In slow heart rates the stroke volume is maintained, but the heart rate is reduced. Simple maths calculates that this will have a reductive impact on cardiac output. Depending on the cause, slow heart rates can deteriorate into complete stoppage of the heart, asystole or an uncoordinated ventricular rhythm such as ventricular fibrillation. Conversely when the heart rate is too fast, the heart is not given opportunity to fill before the next beat is initiated. This means that when the heart beats, it is beating 'half empty'. This reduces stroke volume and cardiac output is reduced despite the fast rate. Fast heart rates are tiring for the heart to maintain for any great length of time. They produce a poor cardiac output in spite of a tremendous amount of energy being invested. They can quickly exhaust the heart and lead to cardiac arrest. Some of these fast rhythms will spontaneously revert to a more normal rhythm without treatment.

In uncoordinated rhythms, the lack of organisation prevents a normal beat being orchestrated and as such these rhythms are incapable of producing a good quality cardiac output. They may produce no output at all. Where no cardiac output is produced, the person is said to be in cardiac arrest. The most important of these uncoordinated rhythms is ventricular fibrillation. Here the heart essentially wobbles like a jelly and is unable to pump blood. Ventricular fibrillation is a cardiac arrest rhythm that needs immediate treatment with cardiopulmonary resuscitation and electrical defibrillation.

Managing arrhythmias

The management of arrhythmias in the initial stages largely centres on rate control. The strategies that are employed involve speeding up a slow heart, slowing a fast heart and restoring order to an uncoordinated heart. These aims are achieved by using drugs or electrical therapies. Important drugs of note are:

- Atropine, which is used to speed up the heart rate
- Adenosine, which is used to slow the heart rate
- Beta-blockers, which are used to slow the heart rate
- Digoxin, which slows conduction in the heart
- Amiodarone, which increases the length of time it takes the heart to beat.

Electrical therapies

Electrical therapies can be used to restore order, slow the heart and increase the heart rate. The options for electrical treatment of arrhythmias are basically pacemakers, cardioversion and defibrillation. Knowledge of the cardiac anatomy and the nature of arrhythmias is required in order to understand how these therapies function. For a fuller discussion of the electrical therapies see Chapter 6.

Failure of the valves in the heart

In health, blood flows through the heart in one direction. A series of valves serves to ensure that this unidirectional blood flow is maintained. Damage to or failure of the valves can reduce the effectiveness of the heart, impairing and sometimes arresting cardiac output. The main problems that can occur with the valves in the heart are:

- They were never functional (congenital problems)
- They developed a growth, preventing normal function (such as in endocarditis)
- They become hardened and narrowed (stenosis)
- Their leaflets allow back flow of blood (regurgitation)
- The muscle holding the valve leaflets in place ruptures, rendering the valve useless.

There is little that can be done to resolve valve problems without expert surgical or radiological assistance and so any further discussion is beyond the scope of this chapter.

Damage to the sac around the heart

The heart is contained in a double-layered fibrous sac known as the pericardium. Between the layers exists a potential space referred to as the pericardial cavity. In health the pericardial cavity is filled with a small volume of serous fluid that facilitates the movement of the heart as it contracts. A further function of the pericardium is to prevent the heart from over-distending during diastolic filling. The pericardium prevents over-distension of the heart by providing only a limited amount of space for the heart to expand into.

Certain illness states can result in a collection of fluid or blood forming in the pericardium (pericardial effusion). This in turn limits the amount of space available in which the heart can distend, thus reducing the amount of blood that can fill the heart during the diastolic phase of the cardiac cycle. Cardiac tamponade develops where the collection of fluid in the pericardium becomes so great that the heart can no longer effectively fill and as a result the cardiac output is reduced. If this progresses rapidly, it can result in cardiac arrest.

Patients with pericardial tamponade can be recognised from a group of three symptoms referred to as Beck's triad: muffled heart sounds on auscultation, distended neck veins and hypotension. Treatment of pericardial tamponade is by aspiration of the fluid that has collected in the pericardium. This is performed by a technique called pericardiocentesis. In an emergency, pericardiocentesis can be performed using a large-bore (14-gauge) cannula, attached to a 50-mL syringe connected via a 3-way tap. This is then inserted into the chest 2 cm below the xiphoid process at a 45-degree angle, aiming towards the left shoulder. The cannula is advanced while watching the ECG monitor screen. When an injury pattern is seen on the ECG (ST segment elevation) the needle is withdrawn slightly and the effusion aspirated. The wider availability of ultrasound now means that pericardiocentesis can be guided by ultrasound when both the equipment and trained operators are available. Occasionally, the effusion may be too viscous to be aspirated through the cannula and urgent surgery will be needed to decompress the pericardium. Special pericardiocentesis kits do exist, although they may not always be available.

Cardiac function can also be impaired by constrictive pericarditis. This is more of a progressive condition in which the pericardium thickens and tightens around the heart, restricting diastolic filling. Treatment for this condition is surgical.

Blood volume

When the volume of blood in the body is reduced, the person is said to be hypovolaemic. Hypovolaemia is the most common cause of shock and should always be considered first in any shocked patient in the absence of any other obvious cause. There are two mechanisms that lead to the development of hypovolaemia. The first is direct loss of blood and the second is a lack of total fluid in the body (dehydration). Blood loss, leading to hypovolaemia can be either internal or external and the absence of obvious external blood loss should be no reassurance to the absence of hypovolaemia. Where blood loss is the cause of the hypovolaemia, stemming any further loss is a priority over the replacement of fluids. Ideally, the actions should be performed concurrently. Where the blood loss is external, direct pressure should be applied and the wound elevated above the level of the heart if this is possible. If a foreign object remains in the wound, no pressure should be applied over this and dressings should be applied at the sides of the object. Where the bleeding is internal, surgery or an interventional radiological procedure may be required to arrest the flow of blood.

Dehydration, leading to hypovolaemic shock, can occur as a result of prolonged periods of vomiting, diarrhoea or excessive sweating. Body fluid can also be lost via wound exudates and this is a particular problem in people with serious burn injuries. High urine output states are another important cause of hypovolaemia as they precipitate dehydration. An excessive urine output is a feature of hyperglycaemia in the patient with poorly treated diabetes mellitus. Patients with diabetes insipidus and high output renal failure are also at risk of dehydration. Failure to drink sufficient quantities of fluids, particularly during times of illness, is an additional, yet important, cause of shock that should not be overlooked.

The treatment for hypovolaemia involves replacing fluid. There are several types of fluid that can be used but the exact fluid remains debated. The two main types of fluid that are available to replace lost volume can be grouped into crystalloids and colloids.

The crystalloids are fluids such as sodium chloride solution 0.9%, Hartmann's solution and 5% dextrose solution. These are relatively inert substances and can be used safely to replace lost fluid. Crystalloids quickly diffuse out of the blood into the interstitial space. This has the advantage of replacing fluid lost from the tissues. The disadvantage is that several units of crystalloid must be given to replace a single unit of lost blood.

Colloid solutions, such as Haemaccel and Gelofusine, have a higher molecular weight than the crystalloids. This provides the colloids with the ability to remain in the intravascular space for longer than crystalloids. While this is useful for the initial management of blood loss, it does not replace fluid loss from the tissues. Colloids are also more expensive than crystalloids. They have the ability to provoke allergic reaction, and they contain other components such as potassium, making them unsuitable for some individuals. Consensus of opinion supports crystalloids, such as sodium chloride 0.9%, as safe and effective solutions for the replacement of fluid in the early stages of management of the acutely ill.

Intravenous fluid therapy is used in two main ways. The first is to provide maintenance fluids for the person who is not able to drink sufficient amounts in order to maintain normal homeostatic balance. The second is to rapidly replace blood volume and body fluid when the person has lost circulating volume or is dehydrated.

Maintenance fluids

To identify if a person requires maintenance fluids, it is necessary to calculate the amount of fluid that the patient requires in a 24-hour period. In order to do this, Cooper et al. (2006) have proposed a formula to use. They calculate, as a minimum, patients require:

- 4 mL/kg for the first 10 kg of weight
- 2 mL/kg for the second 10 kg of weight
- 1 mL/kg for each kg of weight after that.

This formula calculates the amount of fluid that a person needs per hour. To establish the basic fluid requirement per day, the volume calculated in the above formula needs to be multiplied by 24. Once the basic fluid requirement has been calculated, the need for maintenance fluids can be identified and titrated against fluid balance charts. The protocol that should be followed to do this is illustrated in Figure 5.4. It is necessary to recognise that this provides a guide only and individual patient assessment

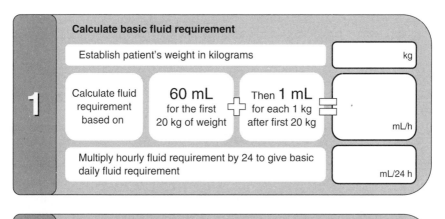

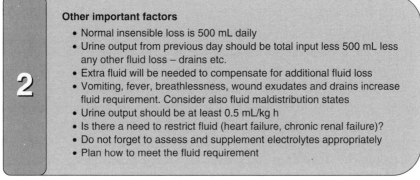

FIGURE 5.4   *Protocol for calculating fluid requirements.*

is needed to dictate the type of fluid and the need for supplementation with potassium.

Rapid volume replacement

When a patient is volume-deficient, a fluid challenge can be given to restore the lost volume. Giving a fluid challenge involves giving a bolus of fluid, usually 500 mL rapidly. The administration of a fluid challenge should be goal directed. Signs of compensation for volume depletion should trigger the administration of a fluid challenge. After each challenge the patient should be reassessed. Challenges should be repeated until a response is seen. A response is defined as an improvement or reversal of the signs that indicate that a compensatory mechanism has been activated. If no response is seen then consider an alternative cause for the patient's condition.

The administration of large amounts of fluid to patients is not without risk and caution needs to be exercised so as not to induce heart failure, create a fluid overloaded state or damage any blood clots that have already formed and are preventing further blood loss. In patients with known heart failure or signs of new heart failure, renal impairment or in the very elderly, the volume of fluid used to provide a challenge should be reduced to 250 mL and the patient's condition re-evaluated after each bolus is given, looking specifically for signs of worsening heart failure, fluid overload, as well as improvements in the volume status of the patient.

Administering too much fluid to a patient can cause fluid overload (hypervolaemia). This produces symptoms similar to heart failure and you should be mindful of this in your patients who have received fluid. Patients who are victims of trauma or those who have recently undergone surgery also need special consideration when it comes to intravenous fluid therapy. After an injury, the body forms blood clots to naturally stem bleeding. These blood clots are not as robust as the healthy tissue that normally occupies this space. The lower blood pressure that occurs after injury facilitates blood clots to stem the flow of blood. If blood pressure is returned to normal, any clots that have formed may be ruptured by the increase in blood pressure. A strategy has been developed to avoid this problem and is termed permissive hypotension. This works on the principle that patients with trauma and who have become hypotensive should only be given fluids titrated to maintain a blood pressure of 90–100 mmHg systolic. This limits damage to forming blood clots and reduces the risk of re-bleeding.

Peripheral vascular resistance

The final aspect of the perfusion triad that needs to be discussed is that of peripheral vascular resistance. Understanding the role that vascular resistance plays in maintaining perfusion requires an appreciation of the permeability of blood vessels and the amount of muscular tone the vessels hold. The patency of the blood vessels is also essential for maintaining perfusion.

Capillary permeability

The capillaries are semipermeable blood vessels. In health, a limit is placed on the amount of fluid leaking out of the capillaries into the interstitial space. At time of illness, inflammation of the capillary can lead to extra fluid leaking out of the capillary into the interstitial space. This is an important mechanism that helps the body to deal with local tissue damage. When inflammation is widespread, large volumes of fluid are lost from the intravascular space into the interstitial space. This is a phenomenon called fluid maldistribution and is a feature of shock caused by anaphylaxis (severe allergy) and sepsis (severe infection). This also occurs in systemic inflammatory response syndrome (SIRS). Fluid maldistribution can also occur when fluid leaks from the intravascular space into a space within the body that does not usually contain fluid. When this occurs, it is referred to as the third space. Examples of the third space include the collection of fluid in the peritoneum, which occurs with liver disease, and pancreatitis.

Systemic vascular resistance

Blood vessels are able to dilate and constrict. This ability assists the body to regulate blood pressure and temperature and deal with illness states. In health, regulation of the amount of constriction and dilation is governed by nervous innervation of the smooth muscle that lines blood vessels and the amount of vasoactive chemical messengers in the blood that are either pro-dilation or pro-constriction. If one of these mechanisms fails or becomes overzealous, then either dilation or constriction will predominate. We have already seen that when inflammation occurs, capillaries become more permeable, allowing extra fluid to leak from the intravascular space into the interstitial space. As part of the inflammatory response, chemicals such as histamine are released locally. Histamine promotes dilation of the blood vessels. When histamine is released locally it dilates the blood vessel, which assists the immune response, allowing white cells an opportunity to access damaged tissue. Where histamine release is widespread it causes widespread dilation, reducing blood pressure and is a second mechanism that leads to shock from an allergic or infectious cause.

Sepsis and septic shock are serious conditions that have been associated with poor patient outcome. To challenge this situation the Surviving Sepsis Campaign has produced an international guideline which draws together all of the best science in how to identify and manage patients with these conditions (see Further reading).

Important steps in the management of anaphylaxis involve recognising the condition and the rapid administration of intramuscular adrenaline at a dose of 0.5 mg. Again, specific guidance exists on the management of anaphylaxis (see Further reading).

The diameter of blood vessels is also influenced by the sympathetic nervous system. This innervation causes constriction and dilation of the larger muscular vessels in order to maintain blood pressures at an acceptable level. In patients who experience a serious insult to the brain or spinal cord, this normal function of the sympathetic nervous system is removed and blood vessels can dilate in an unopposed manner. This results in blood pooling in the peripheral vasculature and not circulating, reducing the effective circulating volume and causing shock. This type of shock is different from the other types as it is characterised by a lack of sympathetic activity. Bradycardia is common as is a full bounding pulse with a narrow pulse pressure.

Shock caused by increased permeability and dilation of the blood vessels is not usually responsive to fluid therapy alone. Fluids can, when given, simply leak out into the interstitial space and pool in the dilated vessels. Here vasopressors and possibly inotropic drugs are also required. These drugs act to restore effective circulation with vasopressors bringing about vasoconstriction and inotropes increasing the strength of the heart's contractions. Noradrenaline is an example of a vasopressor drug and dobutamine is an example of an inotrope. Both inotropes and vasopressors used in the management of shock are given by infusion. Their use is usually restricted to patients receiving critical care as they need to be titrated against physiological response. This can be reliably monitored only by using invasive monitoring devices available in the critical care setting. Like all drugs, vasopressors and inotropes can cause problems when used inappropriately. High doses of vasopressors intended to raise blood pressure can cause ischaemic damage to peripheral structures. They also increase the workload of the heart, which can be detrimental to circulation. As their use is relatively complex, they should only be used by people trained and experienced in their administration.

Obstruction to the flow of blood is the third and final consideration when considering the health of blood vessels. In obstructive shock there is a normal blood volume. The problem here is that blood cannot circulate properly, due to a physical obstruction to blood flow. Classically, the most common cause of this condition is massive pulmonary embolism. A massive pulmonary embolism blocks blood vessels in the lungs preventing blood from passing from the right side to the left side of the heart. This in turn results in no blood being available for the left side of the heart to pump, quickly resulting in a profoundly shocked patient. In some patients, the first sign of this may be cardiac arrest, where there is complete absence of blood flow. Treatment of pulmonary embolisms depends on the size, location and risk factors. The basic treatment is anticoagulation with low molecular weight heparin. Thrombolysis or embolectomy are alternative management strategies for larger emboli. Prevention of venous thromboembolism (VTE) is an important consideration in all hospitalised patients, especially those undergoing surgery or those with malignant disease. Prophylactic heparin and anti-embolic stockings are important, commonly used strategies to prevent VTE. Patients at particular risk of VTE can be fitted with an inferior vena cava filter to prevent thrombi reaching the heart and subsequently embolising in the lungs.

Conclusion

The maintenance of an effective circulation depends on many factors. Each of the components that contribute to maintaining circulation has a specific role to play and, should it become disordered, the circulation can fail to a greater or lesser degree. Circulatory disorders which cause shock are classified according to cause. The medical management of shock is directed at correcting the cause of the shock. This chapter provided an overview of some of the most important types of shock and the strategies used to manage them were outlined in brief. This has been done in order to promote a global understanding of how circulation fails. Motivated readers will want to augment the information presented here with some more detailed reading into the specific causes of shock and their management. Suggested texts are included in the Further reading section of this chapter.

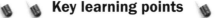

Key learning points

- The circulation of blood provides an essential transport system for oxygen and nutrients.
- Systemic failure of the circulation is called shock.
- Shock results in inadequate delivery of oxygen to the tissues and a removal of waste products.
- Shock can be caused by a lack of blood, poor heart function, obstruction to blood flow or maldistribution of fluid within the body.
- The causes of shock are summarised by the perfusion triad.
- Shock seriously upsets homeostasis and in serious cases can directly cause death.
- Treatment for shock is to restore normal circulatory function.
- Options for the management of shock are directed by its cause.

Self-assessment questions

1 Which of the following is not a part of the perfusion triad?

   A   Cardiac pump
   B   Blood volume
   C   Peripheral vascular resistance
   D   Potassium content

2 Which of the following is not a classification of shock?

   A   Hypovolaemic
   B   Neurogenic
   C   Obstructive
   D   Septic
   E   Compensatory

3 Defibrillation is used to treat which of the following arrhythmias?

   A   Ventricular ectopic
   B   Ventricular fibrillation
   C   Atrial fibrillation
   D   Bradycardia
   E   Asystole

4 Which fluid is the safest to use for the immediate replacement of blood volume?

   A   Glucose 5%
   B   Haemaccel
   C   Dextran
   D   Sodium chloride 0.9%
   E   Sodium chloride 1.45%

5 Which of the following is most important in the management of anaphylaxis?

   A   Colloids
   B   Adrenaline
   C   Glucagon
   D   Sodium chloride
   E   Beta-blockers

6 Beck's triad consist of:

   A   Hypoxia, low oxygen saturation, dyspnoea
   B   Distended neck veins, low blood pressure, tachycardia
   C   Distended neck veins, low blood pressure, muffled heart sounds
   D   Reduced jugular pressure, low blood pressure, muffled heart sounds
   E   Chest pain, shock, cyanosis

7 Vasopressor drugs have what effect on the body?

   A   Increase the contractility of the heart
   B   Reduce the workload of the heart
   C   Stimulate vasoconstriction
   D   Stimulate vasodilation
   E   Reduce oxygen demand

8 The basic 24-hour fluid requirement of an 80-kg man is:

   A   1000 mL
   B   1080 mL
   C   2000 mL
   D   2880 mL
   E   4000 mL

9 What is the aim of giving aspirin to a person with a suspected ACS?

   A   Relieve pain
   B   Suppress inflammation
   C   Dissolve blood clots blocking coronary vessels
   D   Prevent further platelet aggregation
   E   All of the above

10 What is the initial adult dose of adrenaline when given intramuscularly to a patient with anaphylaxis?

   A   0.1 mg
   B   1 mg
   C   200 mg
   D   10 mg
   E   0.5 mg

Answers

1D, 2E, 3B, 4D, 5B, 6C, 7C, 8D, 9D, 10E.

Further reading

Dellinger, R.P., Levy, M.M. and Carlet, J.M., et al. (2008) 'Surviving Sepsis Campaign: International guidelines for management of severe sepsis and septic shock: 2008 [published correction appears in *Crit Care Med* 2008; 36: 1394–1396]', *Critical Care in Medicine* 2008; 36: 296–327.
This is an important updated guideline that provides consensus of opinion on how patients with sepsis and septic shock can be recognised and managed.

Gray, H., Dawkins, K., Morgan, J. and Simpson, I. (2008) *Lecture Notes in Cardiology*. Oxford: Blackwell Publishing.
This text explains the conditions that can affect the heart and blood vessels in greater depth than has been possible here. It is both accessible and authoritative.

Resuscitation Council UK (2008) *Emergency Treatment of Anaphylactic Reactions: Guidelines for Healthcare Providers*. London: Resuscitation Council UK.
This important guideline outlines how to respond to a person with anaphylaxis.

6

Electrocardiographic monitoring

Chapter aims

By the end of this chapter you should be able to:

- Discuss the role of ECG monitoring as part of comprehensive assessment of cardiac function
- Describe the anatomy of the cardiac conduction system and relate this to the ECG
- Explain how the ECG is generated
- List and identify commonly encountered cardiac arrhythmias
- Summarise the types of management used in common cardiac arrhythmias

---

The electrocardiograph or ECG is an important tool used in the monitoring of the acutely ill. It is, however, a tool that is the source of much concern and significant confusion for many health professionals. To become fully conversant with the ECG takes a tremendous amount of commitment, energy and experience, although a basic working understanding can be quickly developed in those who are eager to learn. This chapter will explain some basic concepts about the ECG in order to provide a basis for practice. It is not the intention to address all of the electrocardiographic findings that may be seen in practice, as this would be difficult to include in a single book. Rather, this chapter will concern itself with developing a practitioner's ability to recognise those cardiac rhythms that are relevant to acute illness and require rapid recognition and management.

Definitions

Before one can start to learn about the ECG there are some important
terms that need to be defined. The ECG is a graphical representation of
the electrical activity of the heart. It is created by electrodes placed on the
skin that collect electrical information about how the heart is contracting.
The most diagnostic of ECGs is the 12-lead recording which provides 12
different views of the heart from standardised positions. While this is the
most informative of ECGs and provides information about the morphol-
ogy and rhythm of the heart it requires the placement of ten separate leads
on the patient and is impractical for continuous monitoring. To overcome
this practical problem, systems with three, four and five leads are used to
continually monitor a person's heart when they become acutely ill. This is
called cardiac monitoring and it is the interpretation of the cardiac rhythm
that this chapter will be concerned with. In practice, a combination of
12-lead ECGs and cardiac monitoring is used to provide information
about a patient's cardiac function.

Let us now consider the findings of the ECG. Essentially, when undertaking an ECG you are looking to identify if a person has a normal cardiac
rhythm or an abnormal one. The normal cardiac rhythm is termed normal
sinus rhythm or NSR, and abnormal rhythms are referred to as arrhythmias. Arrhythmia is a collective term that is given to a cardiac rhythm that
is not normal. Some people use the term dysrhythmia to describe abnormal rhythms. However, for the remainder of this text the term arrhythmia
will be used.

Additional terms are used to describe disorders of heart rate regardless
of cause. Again these are umbrella terms that are used to describe rhythms
that are unduly fast or slow. A rhythm is defined as a tachycardia if it is 100
beats per minute (bpm) or more. Bradycardia occurs if the heart rate is 60
or fewer beats per minute. Knowing this fact helps tremendously with
interpreting the cardiac monitor as one can exclude a large number of
rhythms just by considering the heart rate. For example a patient with a
heart rate of 40 bpm can never be described as having any of the
tachycardias.

Anatomy of the cardiac conduction system

The starting point in being able to understand the ECG is to understand
the anatomy of the heart, particularly the cardiac conduction system, as the
ECG only shows what is occurring electrophysiologically within the heart.

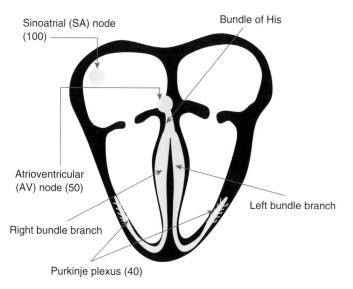

FIGURE 6.1   *Anatomy of the cardiac conduction system with spontaneous discharge rates (per minute) shown in brackets.*

Because of the importance of this anatomical knowledge, you are encouraged to ensure that you fully understand the anatomy before moving on to the next section. Figure 6.1 shows the anatomy of the cardiac conduction system, which consists of:

- The sinoatrial node (SA; the normal cardiac pacemaker)
- The atrioventricular node (AV)
- Bundle of His
- Left bundle branch

  ○ Anterior superior division (fascicle)
  ○ Posterior inferior division (fascicle)

- Right bundle branch
- Purkinje plexus.

The purpose of the cardiac conduction system is to excite or stimulate the myocardial (heart muscles) cells to contract and create a heart beat. In order to do this in a coordinated way, the conduction system must regulate both the order and speed at which myocardial cells are stimulated to contract or an arrhythmia will develop. In the healthy individual, the SA node is the pacemaker (the pacemaker is where the heart beat originates). Discharge in the SA node causes the atria to contract (atrial systole). The atria are electrically isolated or insulated from the ventricles by a fibrous skeleton that prevents the atrial contraction spreading to the ventricles before the atria have finished contracting. In the healthy heart, the only connection between the atria and ventricles is through the AV node. The AV node serves to gather the electrical impulses from the atria and delay the conduction into the ventricles so that the atria can finish contracting completely before the ventricles start to contract. Then, after a short pause (0.12–0.20 seconds, equivalent to three to five small squares on the ECG paper) the electrical impulse is rapidly transmitted down the bundle of His into the left and right bundle branches and onto the Purkinje fibres, causing the ventricles to contract.

If the SA node fails to initiate an impulse, or initiates impulses too slowly, each lower part of the conduction system has the ability to self-initiate a contraction in a sort of back-up mechanism. Rhythms that arise as a result of a delayed impulse will normally be slower than rhythms that originate from the SA node. Figure 6.1 gives the spontaneous discharge rates of different parts of the cardiac conduction system. When the heart beat originates from any place other than the SA node, the focus of the beat's origin is said to be an ectopic or abnormal pacemaker site.

Formation of electrical current and the ECG

The next step in understanding the ECG is to translate the electrical impulse that passes through the heart into a graphical representation so that it can be assessed.

Cells of the heart, in a resting (non-beating) state are said to be polarised. A polarised cell is one that has potassium (K) and sodium (Na) ions on opposite sides of the cell membrane. K preferentially exists within the cell and Na without. When stimulated by an electrical impulse from the conducting system, K is allowed to leak out of the cell and Na is allowed to leak in. This process is called depolarisation and occurs as myocardial cells contract, creating a heart beat. When cells are in a depolarised state they are unable to be stimulated and contract again until the equilibrium between Na and K has been re-established. Tiny chemical pumping stations on the cell membrane constantly pump Na out of the cells and K into the cells to ensure the correct balance. When a cell has been depolarised and is refractory to stimulation these tiny Na and K pumps restore the balance so that Na is held outside the cell and K inside the cell. This process is called repolarisation (Figure 6.2).

The shift of Na and K across the cell membrane generates a small electrical current that is detected on the surface of the skin by special

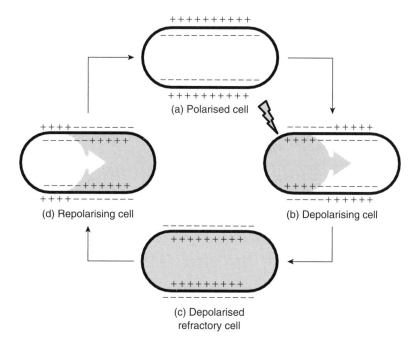

FIGURE 6.2 *Contraction of myocardial cells: (a) differential inter– and extracellular potassium and sodium ion concentrations set up a resting potential difference across the cell membrane. (b) Electrical stimulation from the conductive system causes movement of sodium and potassium in and out of the cell. (c) Once fully depolarised, the cell cannot contract again. (d) Small pumps in the cell membrane restore sodium and potassium to their original concentrations and a small electrical potential is restored.*

electrodes and displayed on the ECG monitor screen. As the heart is a complex shape, electrodes placed on different places on the chest wall will show a different pattern of electrical activity despite looking at the same heart. The scientific reasons for this are basic, yet beyond the scope of this chapter. However, this is the reason why 12-lead ECGs provide more information than the simple three-lead monitor.

In ECG monitoring, the electrodes are usually placed on the patient's chest, although the leads that are used to acquire the electrical image are formally considered to be limb leads (the leads that are usually placed on the limbs when acquiring a 12-lead ECG). The leads can then be placed on either the chest or the limbs to achieve a satisfactory image. When monitoring a patient over time, having the leads connected to the limbs can limit activity, so attaching the leads to the chest can be more convenient. Box 6.1 provides guidelines on how to position ECG electrodes on the chest. In a simple three-lead assembly the red electrode can be attached to the patient's right clavicle, the yellow electrode to the left clavicle and the green or black electrode on the last rib in the anterior axillary line.

BOX 6.1   Positioning ECG electrodes for cardiac monitoring

- Position electrodes remotely from defibrillation sites
- Position electrodes over bone not muscle
- Shave chest hair if necessary
- Wipe area with alcohol swab (especially if patient is sweaty) – do not use alcohol before applying defibrillation pacing pads or if the patient is likely to require defibrillation imminently
- Do not position electrodes over burned skin

The connection of the right arm, left arm and foot leads produce a triangle around the heart known as Einthoven's triangle (Figure 6.3). Willem Einthoven was Dutch doctor who first pioneered the development and use of electrocardiography. He invented a system that required the limbs to be placed in buckets of water in order to detect the electrical current generated by the heart. This conformation effectively produces a triangle around the heart with the shoulders and the groin being the points on the triangle. The connection between the right arm and left arm electrodes produces a view of the heart known as lead I. Connections between the right arm and the foot lead produce a view of the heart known as lead II. Finally connection between the left arm and the foot lead is described as lead III. These different leads simply represent different views of the electrical activity of the heart, and their locations are illustrated in Figure 6.3.

The ECG monitor, if not connected to a patient, will show a flat line called the isoelectric line. Once a patient is connected, if one is looking at the heart from lead II, a common monitoring lead, then any electrical current travelling towards the electrode will create a positive (upward going) deflection on the ECG such as the P, R and T waves. If the current is travelling away from the monitor, then a negative (downward going) deflection will be seen such as the Q and S waves (Figure 6.4).

The normal ECG

As mentioned above, the normal cardiac rhythm is referred to as the normal sinus rhythm (NSR). For rhythm to be classified as sinus, the ECG

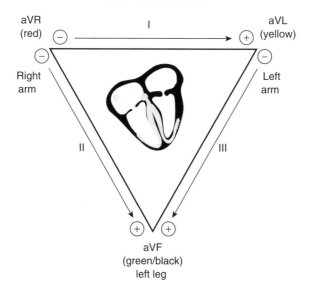

FIGURE 6.3 *Einthoven triangle showing the position of electrodes and the views of the heart seen by each monitoring lead.*

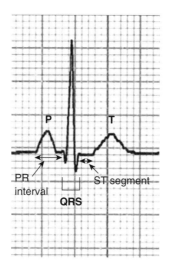

FIGURE 6.4 *The normal ECG complex with waveforms labelled. P, atrial contraction; PR interval (shown by arrow), pause at the AV node; QRS, ventricular contraction; T, ventricular repolarisation.*

must show normal depolarisation and repolarisation in an ordered fashion at an acceptable rate. The normal ECG complex is shown in Figure 6.4. This graphical representation of electrical activity in the heart is directly related to the systematic depolarisation and repolarisation of myocardial cells. Atrial contraction (depolarisation) is triggered by a discharge from the SA node and is represented on the ECG by the creation of a P wave. The delay that occurs at the AV node causes a short period where the ECG complex returns to the isoelectric line – this is referred to as the PR interval. Following this pause at the AV node, the electrical impulse is rapidly conducted through the AV node to the bundle of His and to the left and right bundle branches, causing a QRS complex to be seen on the ECG monitor as ventricular contraction occurs. Repolarisation of the ventricles is shown by the T wave. Repolarisation of the atria creates only a small current and as it occurs at the same time as ventricular depolarisation is often obscured by the QRS complex but can become obvious in tachycardia as a Ta wave.

Blood flow and the ECG

In the healthy heart, the electrical activity directly relates to the mechanical activity. When the myocardial cell depolarises, an electrical current is generated at the same time that the cell contracts, propelling blood though the heart. It follows then that if there is an abnormality in the ECG, there is likely to be abnormality with the mechanical activity of the heart. This mechanical abnormality in turn impairs blood flow through the heart – making the heart's function less than optimal, possibly reducing cardiac output. In the healthy heart, when the SA node initiates a heart beat, the atria are filled with blood, so when a P wave is seen atrial contraction is occurring, which empties the full atria into the ventricles. Then the PR interval allows the atria to empty completely into the ventricles before the QRS complex is seen, signalling ventricular contraction, and with it emptying the ventricles into the pulmonary artery and aorta. When the T wave is seen, there is atrial filling occurring ready for the next impulse from the SA node, which will trigger the cycle to be repeated.

It follows then that if there is a problem with the electrical conduction in the heart such as an arrhythmia, there is likely to be a problem to a greater or lesser degree with blood flow. In turn, blood pressure and organ perfusion may be affected, resulting in a disestablishment of homeostasis. It is possible to discern what the problem with blood flow is by considering the ECG. For example, if there are no P waves, there will be no active ventricular filling and an inefficient heart beat will occur. Table 6.1 summarises common problems that can occur with blood flow based on ECG findings. Probably the most notable exception to normal functioning of the heart occurs when the person has a type of cardiac arrest called pulseless electrical activity (PEA). In PEA there is electrical activity seen on the

TABLE 6.1 *Arrhythmias and how they can cause problems with blood flow*

Cardiac rhythm	Blood flow disorder
Tachycardias • Sinus tachycardia • Narrow complex tachycardia • Broad complex tachycardia	In general, rapid heart rates allow little time for diastolic filling. This results in the heart beating while inadequately filled effectively and pumping while half empty. Thus the heart invests a lot of effort to circulate little blood. Tachycardias also increase the oxygen demand of the heart as it is working harder, which requires more energy. Broad complex tachycardia can be a cardiac arrest rhythm
Sinus bradycardia	Heart rate too slow to move sufficient blood
Heart blocks • Second degree heart block type 1 • Second degree heart block type 2 • Third degree heart block	Ventricles occasionally fail to receive the electrical stimulation needed to trigger a contraction. No output from the ventricles for that beat. If this occurs too often, cardiac output will be compromised. In third degree heart block there is total dissociation between the atria and ventricles. This causes a potentially serious abnormality where the atria may try to empty into full ventricles and the ventricles may attempt to contract when empty. Can precipitate a serious reduction in cardiac output
Atrial fibrillation	Uncoordinated atrial fibrillation (wobbling) leads to uncoordinated passive ventricular filling. This in turn leads to a variable stroke volume
Ventricular fibrillation	Uncoordinated ventricular wobbling leads to an absence of cardiac output
Asystole	Total absence of electrical activity in the heart results in no ventricular contraction, thus producing no cardiac output
Pulseless electrical activity	Electrical activity from which one would normally expect to feel a pulse, but with the absence of blood flow there is no cardiac output

monitor that is normally associated with a perfusing rhythm; however, in PEA no cardiac output is generated and no pulse is felt – hence the name of this phenomenon. In PEA the heart may well still be contracting and the reason for the absence of a cardiac output can most commonly be accounted for as a result of an absence of blood to pump in profound hypovolaemia, or some sort of mechanical compression of the heart that prevents it from either filling during diastole or emptying during systole.

Normal sinus rhythm

The normal rhythm of the heart is called normal sinus rhythm as it originates from the sinus node. For the rhythm to be sinus there must be ordered conduction down the normal conduction pathway with a regular heart rate from 61 to 99 bpm. Figure 6.5 shows an example of normal sinus rhythm.

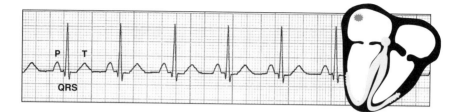

FIGURE 6.5   *Normal sinus rhythm. Pacemaker is SA with a rate of 61–99 beats per minute.*

Problems with cardiac rhythm – arrhythmias

Patients can experience a wide range of arrhythmias, and some of the most commonly seen are explained in this chapter. To aid you in identifying the abnormalities of cardiac rhythm, the basic characteristics of each arrhythmia are explained. Like the need to understand the conduction system before attempting to interpret the ECG, it is also important to have an understanding of all the potential arrhythmias as efforts at ECG interpretation require an understanding of the potential diagnosis before one can succeed. The ECG changes seen can be subtle or dramatic, yet both types of change can require immediate intervention if lives are to be saved. Box 6.2 shows a list of common rhythms encountered in practice.

BOX 6.2   Potential cardiac rhythms and arrhythmias in practice

- Normal sinus rhythm
- Sinus tachycardia
- Sinus bradycardia
- Sinus arrhythmia
- Sinus arrest
- Narrow complex tachycardia
- Broad complex tachycardia
- First degree heart block
- Second degree heart block type 1
- Second degree heart block type 2
- Third degree heart block
- Atrial fibrillation
- Atrial flutter
- Ventricular fibrillation
- Asystole
- Pulseless electrical activity

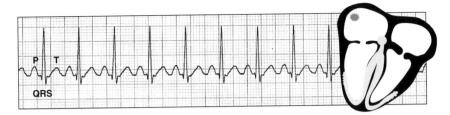

FIGURE 6.6   *Sinus tachycardia: 120 beats per minute. Pacemaker is SA with a rapid rate of discharge >100.*

Sinus tachycardia

Sinus tachycardia is a normal variant of the heart rate at times of stress and exercise. It may also signal a compensation for blood volume loss in the acutely ill. In sinus tachycardia, the pacemaker site of the heart is the SA node and conduction progresses normally down the AV node into the Bundle of His and onto the left and right bundle branches and Purkinje fibres. The ECG complex is essentially normal although it can appear squashed up to the previous complex. The only difference is a heart rate above 100 bpm. Occasionally P waves will be sat on the previous T wave yet be still visible when looked for. Figure 6.6 provides an example of sinus tachycardia.

Sinus bradycardia

Sinus bradycardia is a relatively simple rhythm to diagnose as there exists lots of space in between the ECG complexes, making assessment of slow rhythms relatively easy. Like in sinus tachycardia, the pacemaker site in sinus bradycardia is the SA node and conduction progresses normally down the AV node into the Bundle of His and onto the left and right bundle branches and Purkinje fibres. This normal progression produces a normal looking ECG complex. The difference is that in sinus bradycardia, the heart rate is 60 beats per minute or less. Figure 6.7 provides an example of sinus bradycardia. Symptomatic bradycardia or bradycardias associated with adverse signs or a risk of asystole (see Box 6.4 below) can be treated initially with atropine sulphate. Bradycardias that are not responsive to atropine may require pacing.

Sinus arrhythmia

Sinus arrhythmia is an interesting rhythm variation where there is a normal SA node pacemaker with normal conduction progressing down the AV node into the Bundle of His onto the left and right bundle branches

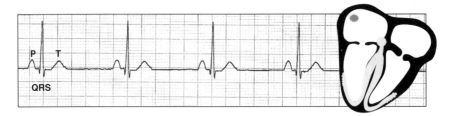

FIGURE 6.7   *Sinus bradycardia. Pacemaker is SA with a slow discharge rate of <60 beats per minute.*

and Purkinje fibres, thus creating a normal-looking ECG complex. Sinus arrhythmia differs from NSR in that the SA node discharges at a variable rate, commonly altering with inspiration and expiration. This can be a normal variant in the young, yet may signify a cardiac pathology in older patients especially if not linked to respiratory pattern.

Narrow complex tachycardia

The term narrow complex tachycardia is an umbrella term used to describe arrhythmias that are thought to originate above the ventricles. These narrow complex tachycardias are sometimes referred to as supraventricular tachycardias (SVTs). While both these terms are not truly a diagnosis in their own right, they do provide a satisfactory description of the arrhythmia for use by novice interpreters. Those with more developed skills and experience in ECG interpretation will be able to sub-classify these rhythms with more accuracy, successfully pinpointing a diagnosis.

The difficulty in pinpointing the diagnosis in narrow complex tachycardias is the rapid rate. This causes the different waves of the ECG complex to be pushed close together making rhythm recognition difficult. Narrow complex tachycardias are, however, likely to be supraventricular as the QRS complex looks normal, suggesting that conduction down the AV node, Bundle of His, and the left and right bundle branches is normal. The use of vagal manoeuvres such as carotid sinus massage or drugs such as adenosine can help to slow the arrhythmia and assist in diagnosis although these should only be used by those specifically trained and experienced in their use. Figure 6.8 gives an example of a narrow complex tachycardia.

Broad complex tachycardia

Broad complex tachycardias are dangerous arrhythmias and can occur in the context of cardiac arrest. Some patients, however, may have a pulse

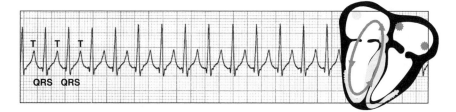

FIGURE 6.8   *Narrow complex tachycardia (supraventricular tachycardia SVT): 180 beats per minute. Note P waves may be present but they become difficult to appreciate as a result of the rapid rate and can be obscured by other larger complexes. Pacemaker site may be SA or could be one or more other supraventricular sites. Occasionally a re-entry circuit may be the cause where energy cycles around the heart.*

despite the presence of a broad complex tachycardia, although there is a risk that the pulse may disappear as the heart tires, resulting in cardiac arrest. Broad complex tachycardia is an umbrella term for all fast rhythms with a broad QRS complex (>0.12 seconds, three small squares on the ECG paper). Like narrow complex tachycardia, broad complex tachycardia is not a diagnosis in its own right and experts can sub-classify the rhythm further. An important cause of broad complex tachycardia is Ventricular tachycardia (VT). In VT the normal SA pacemaker is lost and the rhythm originates from an abnormal ectopic focus within the ventricles. As conduction does not follow the normal pathways, it takes longer to spread across the heart and hence causes a broad or wide QRS complex as shown in Figure 6.9. VT is a malignant rhythm and needs to be managed rapidly due to its association with cardiac arrest. Patients with pulseless VT should be treated as patients with a shockable cardiac arrest rhythm.

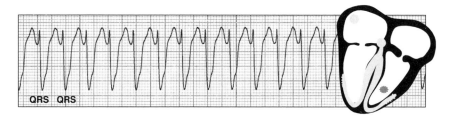

FIGURE 6.9   *Broad complex tachycardia. The QRS is wider than three small squares, 0.12 seconds. This occurs as a result of an ectopic ventricular pacemaker or a block in conduction.*

Ventricular fibrillation

In ventricular fibrillation (VF), there is a loss of the normal SA node pacemaker. Multiple ventricular pacemakers mechanically cause the ventricles to wobble uselessly and produce no palpable cardiac output. VF is always a cardiac arrest rhythm and is treated most successfully with excellent quality cardiopulmonary resuscitation (CPR) and rapid defibrillation. The ECG in VF shows a disorganised, chaotic pattern. At the onset of VF, the waveform can be quite coarse as shown in Figure 6.10a but over a period of time the fibrillatory waves become finer (Figure 6.10b) until the rhythm eventually converts to asystole.

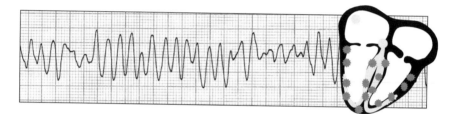

FIGURE 6.10a *Ventricular fibrillation (coarse). Uncoordinated electrical activity seen at a rapid rate with no recognisable QRS complexes – always a cardiac arrest rhythm. Multiple ventricular pacemakers make the heart wobble in an uncoordinated fashion.*

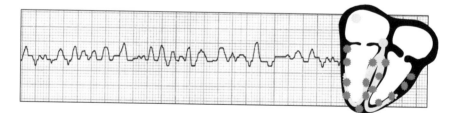

FIGURE 6.10b *Ventricular fibrillation (fine). Same uncoordinated electrical activity as in Figure 6.10a. The amplitude of the wave is reduced; this occurs as the heart tires. It is a later feature of the rhythm and is a precursor to asystole if not treated successfully.*

Atrial fibrillation

Atrial fibrillation (AF) is characterised by a loss of the normal SA node pacemaker. In its place are multiple atrial pacemakers firing at a rate of 300–600 per minute. Obviously if all of these were transmitted to the ventricles there would be a significant tachycardia that would not allow

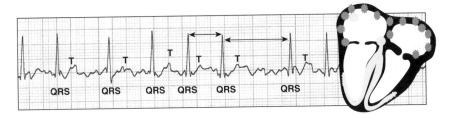

FIGURE 6.11   *Atrial fibrillation (AF). Very irregular rhythm with multiple atrial pacemakers, hence a lack of organised P waves; these are replaced by multiple fibrillatory waves. Not to be confused with ventricular fibrillation as AF is not a cardiac arrest rhythm – unless it is associated with pulseless electrical activity.*

any time for diastolic filling and the patient would undoubtedly suffer haemodynamically. Thankfully, though, the AV node blocks the majority of atrial impulses and only allows a limited number through to excite the ventricles and cause ventricular contraction. On the ECG the loss of SA node activity is seen as a loss of P waves. These are replaced by a large number of irregularly shaped and sized fibrillatory waves which appear in between the QRS complexes. The irregular conduction of impulses from the atria to the ventricles across the AV node results in irregularly timed QRS complexes. These QRS complexes do, however, follow the normal conduction pathway—AV node, Bundle of His, left and right bundle branches and on to the Purkinje fibres. As such the width of the QRS is normal. Figure 6.11 provides an example of a typical AF rhythm.

It is worth noting that because the conduction at the AV node is of a variable rate, AF can be slow, normal or, more commonly, fast, sometimes so fast that it is difficult to see fibrillatory waves and it becomes a narrow complex tachycardia. When this occurs, one of the best clues that the rhythm may be AF is that the QRS complexes are irregular. There are many causes of AF and it can present as a paroxysmal, persistent or permanent rhythm. The most worrying problem associated with AF is the risk of embolisation. As the atria are not contracting in an ordered fashion, this results in blood not being pumped actively from the atria into the ventricles. Ventricular filling is therefore passive and allows blood to pool in the atria and form clots. These clots can then pass into the ventricles where they are pumped either into the lungs from the right heart or more commonly around the body from the left heart and cause an embolism.

Conversion of AF to a more normal rhythm should not be attempted when it cannot be demonstrated that the AF is new in onset as this could cause embolisation of a formed clot. An irregular pulse of varying strength is highly suggestive of AF and requires investigation with a 12-lead ECG if the diagnosis has not already been established. The National Collaborating Centre for Chronic Conditions (2006), funded by the National Institute for Health and Clinical Excellence, has produced guidelines for the diagnosis and treatment of AF and readers may find it beneficial to refer to this informative statement of best practice.

Atrial flutter

In atrial flutter a re-entry circuit is established within the atria; this occurs when an SA node impulse bounces back across the atria and causes additional atrial contraction. This ricocheting of electrical activity can occur several times before it is conducted across the AV node and onto the ventricles. The repeated atrial electrical conduction is shown on the ECG as a characteristic sawtooth flutter wave pattern. Normally the AV node blocks a regular number of atrial impulses and creates a regular ventricular rate with a normal appearance to the QRS. Occasionally, there will be varying degrees of block at the AV node and the ventricular rate (the QRS complexes) will become irregular. Depending on the degree of AV block, atrial flutter can be again fast or slow and can lead to narrow complex tachycardia in some patients. Figure 6.12 shows a typical atrial flutter pattern.

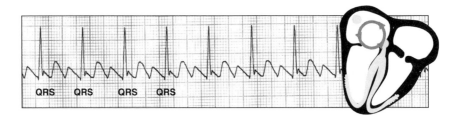

FIGURE 6.12   Atrial flutter. A re-entry circuit is established in the atria. A characteristic sawtooth pattern is seen on the ECG in between the QRS complexes.

Asystole

Asystole or total cardiac asystole is quite possibly one of the simplest arrhythmias to diagnose and is classically associated with romantic and dramatic depictions of death in television dramas. The term asystole quite literally means absence of systole or heart beat. A total absence of electrical activity within the heart is represented on the ECG as a straight, slightly undulating line (Figure 6.13a). It is important to check the presence of

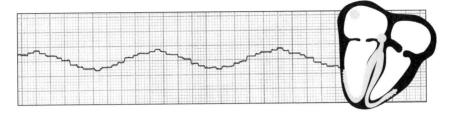

FIGURE 6.13a *Total cardiac asystole. Total absence of electrical activity.*

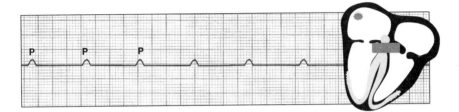

FIGURE 6.13b *Ventricular standstill. P waves present with no ventricular QRS response. This is a type of asystole and will be a cardiac arrest rhythm. The atria contract but conduction is blocked by the AV node. The heart may respond to pacing.*

asystole in two leads to exclude the presence of fine VF which may respond to defibrillation. The presence of asystole on a cardiac monitor is an ominous sign and suggests a poor survival rate, unless there is an obvious reversible cause. Occasionally, asystole with P waves (ventricular standstill) can occur (Figure 6.13b) and this rhythm may respond to pacing.

Heart block

Heart blocks occur when there is a problem in the conduction of the impulse from the atria to the ventricles. This can be due to organic heart disease or chemical imbalances and drug overdose. Some forms of heart block are relatively benign, while others can quickly lead to significant haemodynamic compromise and even cardiac arrest. There are four common types of heart block.

First degree heart block

First degree heart block occurs where there is normal SA node discharge and atrial depolarisation. The problem that occurs is an abnormally long delay at the AV node. This is seen on the ECG as a prolonged PR interval of greater than 0.2 seconds (five small squares on the ECG paper). After

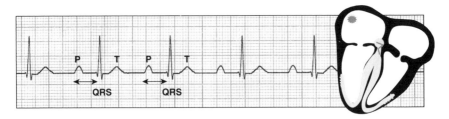

FIGURE 6.14   *First degree heart block. A delay occurs at the AV node, which prolongs the PR interval. The PR interval is measured from the start of the P wave to the start of the QRS complex; it should be no more than five small squares. The long PR interval is shown by the arrows.*

the delay subsides, normal conduction continues and the remainder of the ECG is normal. It can be easy to miss this arrhythmia due to its close resemblance to normal sinus rhythm, so one must have a high index of suspicion if it is to be reliably detected. Figure 6.14 shows an example of first degree heart block. In some patients a mild degree of first degree block may be a normal variant with little clinical significance, although increasing degrees of first degree block warrant investigation.

Second degree heart block type 1

Second degree heart block type 1 or Wenckebach phenomenon is similar to first degree heart block with some important changes. As in first degree heart block, there is a normal SA discharge. This is transmitted to the AV node, where again, like in first degree heart block, there is a delay at the AV junction. The difference that occurs in second degree heart block type 1 is that the delay at the AV junction progressively increases with each beat until a P wave is seen without a QRS following it. A helpful way to remember this arrhythmia is to recall that in Wenckebach phenomenon the P waves 'walk back' from the QRS. Figure 6.15 shows an example of this rhythm.

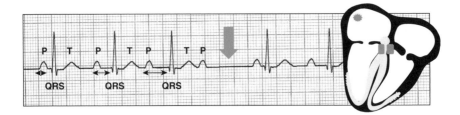

FIGURE 6.15   *Second degree heart block type 1 (Wenckebach phenomenon). Note how the PR interval progressively lengthens until a QRS is not seen (thick arrow). This is an intermittent block at the AV node.*

Second degree heart block type 2

In second degree heart block type 2 there is again a conduction deficit at the AV node. However, here there is no progressive increase in the delay at the AV node. Second degree type 2 is characterised by an intermittent block at the AV node, which results in most of the atrial impulses being conducted normally to the ventricles. Occasionally, there is a total block in conduction at the AV node. On the ECG, this is seen as a normal rhythm with occasional extra normal-looking P waves that are not followed by a QRS complex. Usually this block follows a standard pattern but it can be irregular. Figure 6.16 shows a typical second degree heart block type 2. Second degree heart block type 2 is a risk factor for the development of asystole and requires urgent evaluation.

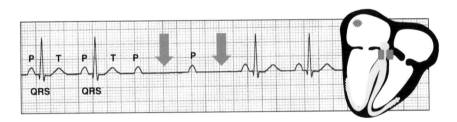

FIGURE 6.16 *Second degree heart block type 2. Intermittent block at the AV node but without progressive lengthening of the PR interval. This rhythm presents a risk of progression to asystole. Non-conducted atrial contraction is shown by a lack of QRS complexes after each P wave (shown by the thick arrows).*

Third degree heart block

Third degree heart block, sometimes referred to as complete heart block, occurs when there is a complete dissociation or block between the activity of the atria and the ventricles. Essentially in third degree AV block the atria and ventricles beat independently of each other. The ECG shows both P waves and QRS complexes, yet there is no identifiable relationship between them. As the QRS originates in the ventricles there is a possibility, depending on the location of its origin, that the QRS will be wider than a normally conducted QRS and this may provide an additional clue to the diagnosis. Complete heart block is a worrying rhythm and has the potential to cause haemodynamic compromise and collapse. Figure 6.17 shows an example of complete heart block.

Pulseless electrical activity

In PEA, you can literally see any rhythm that you would normally expect a pulse from on the ECG, yet clinically there is no palpable pulse.

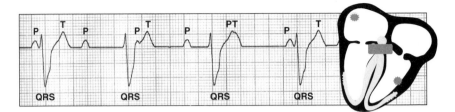

FIGURE 6.17   *Third degree (complete) heart block. Total block at the AV node causes the atria and ventricles to beat independently of each other. There is no relationship between the P waves and QRS complexes. Because of this an additional ventricular pacemaker is seen. Depending on its location, the QRS may appear normal or broad.*

Essentially, the electrical activity of the heart has disassociated itself from the mechanical activity. This can occur when there is a mechanical obstruction to the heart beating or there is no blood for the heart to pump. PEA is always a cardiac arrest rhythm, and requires immediate CPR and identification of its cause followed by appropriate specific management if it is to be successfully reversed. As PEA can present as any rhythm in which one would normally expect to find a pulse, there is little utility in providing an example.

Ectopic and premature beats

To add to the mix, each of the above rhythms can be complicated by ectopic and premature beats. Ectopic beats change the appearance of a rhythm so much and occur commonly that it is important to describe them here and for you to be familiar with them.

Ectopic beats are beats that originate from an abnormal place in the heart. As the SA node is the only place where normal rhythms should originate, technically any beat that originates from a place other than the SA node is classified as ectopic. Ectopic beats are considered as extra beats that are superimposed onto a basic rhythm. A premature beat is a beat that occurs earlier in the cardiac cycle than the next scheduled beat when compared with the remainder of the current heart rhythm. Premature beats either originate from the SA node or have an ectopic focus. When a premature beat occurs from an ectopic focus they are often classified by their place of origin:

- Premature atrial contractions (PACs)
- Premature junctional contractions (PJCs)
- Premature ventricular contractions (PVCs).

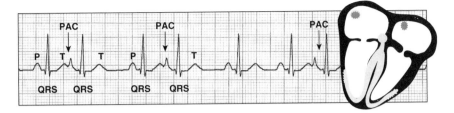

FIGURE 6.18 *Premature atrial contractions (PACs) superimposed on normal sinus rhythm. The PACs (arrowed) show as an abnormally shaped P wave, in this case all followed by a normal looking QRS and T wave.*

PACs are characterised by an extra P wave that is shaped differently from the other P waves. Usually this is followed by a normal QRS. Occasionally though, extra P waves are seen that are not followed by a QRS complex. These can be discriminated from second degree heart block because the P waves are abnormal. Figure 6.18 shows an example of PACs.

PJCs are extra beats that originate somewhere close to the AV junction. They present on the ECG as an extra QRS complex that is not preceded by a P wave. The conduction follows the normal pathway and therefore creates a normal-looking extra QRS complex as shown in Figure 6.19.

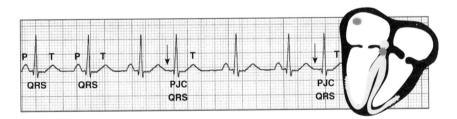

FIGURE 6.19 *Premature junctional contractions (PJC) (arrowed). An extra normal-looking QRS is seen without a preceding P wave.*

Finally, PVCs are extra beats that originate in the ventricles. They are often wide and bizarrely shaped (Figure 6.20a and b). They can originate in one part of the ventricles, 'unifocal' PVCs (Figure 6.20a), or from multiple locations within the ventricles, 'multifocal' PVCs (Figure 6.20b). Occasional unifocal PVCs can be a normal variant, but frequent PVCs or PVCs from multiple sites are concerning and can quickly become unstable, especially if they occur on the T wave of the previous QRS complex (Figure 6.20c), the so called R-on-T phenomenon. In the R-on-T

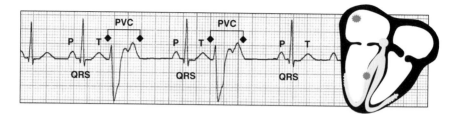

FIGURE 6.20a   *Unifocal premature ventricular contractions (PVC) on sinus rhythm. An extra broad and bizarrely shaped QRS is seen. Each PVC looks the same as it originates from a single focus.*

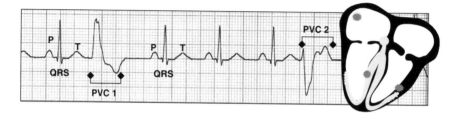

FIGURE 6.20b   *Multifocal premature ventricular contractions (PVC) on sinus rhythm. Two extra broad and bizarrely shaped QRS are seen. Each PVC looks different as it originates from a different part of the heart. A worrying finding.*

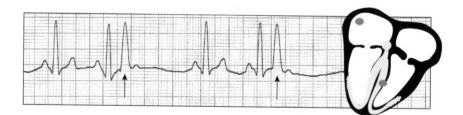

FIGURE 6.20c   *R-on-T premature ventricular contraction. R wave of ectopic beat occurs on the T wave of the previous beat; arrow illustrates the ectopic beat. Can precipitate life-threatening arrhythmia.*

phenomenon, the normal pattern of myocardial repolarisation is interrupted and parts of the heart are then restimulated at this particularly vulnerable time, which can precipitate the development of VF.

Identifying cardiac arrhythmias in practice

Being able to identify a cardiac rhythm requires a good knowledge of the menu of rhythms that could present in practice, as this will allow you to fit what you see on a cardiac monitor with your knowledge of what is going wrong in the heart. Essentially, what you are trying to discover when looking at the ECG rhythm strip is:

1   What is the 'top bit' of the heart doing? (Atrial activity)
2   What is the 'bottom bit' of the heart doing? (Ventricular activity)
3   What is the relationship? (Junctional activity)
4   What is the location of the pacemaker?

To achieve this you need to consider several questions, such as:

1   How fast/slow is the rhythm?
2   Is there a P wave before each QRS?
3   Is there a QRS after every P?
4   Is the rhythm regular or irregular?
5   Is the QRS normal, wide or narrow?

Several things can help you answer these questions successfully. If you are having difficulty in identifying the rhythm on a moving screen, print off a long rhythm strip and assess it on paper. To calculate the rate of the rhythm on paper, count the number of large squares between the R waves and use the information in Box 6.3 to calculate the rate. You can only use this method for regular rhythms.

BOX 6.3   Calculating the heart rate from the number of large squares between the R waves (for use with regular rhythms only)

No of large squares between R waves	Estimated heart rate
1	300
2	150
3	100
4	75
5	60
6	50

Calculating the heart rate for irregular rhythms is a much less accurate activity. A simple method for doing this is to print out ten seconds' (50 large squares) worth of the ECG Strip and then count the number of QRS complexes present. This figure is then multiplied by six to give you an average of the heart rate. It is worth remembering that this is only an estimate and the only way to accurately determine the heart rate in a person with an irregular rhythm is to count all the QRSs that occur over a 60-second period. Even this technique will only confirm the rate for that minute, as subsequent minutes may have different rates depending on the rhythm of the heart. It may then be useful to express the heart rate as a range when there is such variability.

To assist you in drawing conclusions about exactly what rhythm you are looking at, Figure 6.21 provides a simple flowchart that can help you to

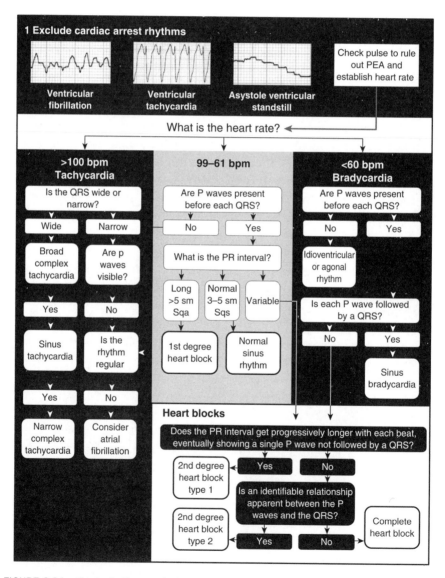

FIGURE 6.21   *Basic rhythm analysis chart.*

identify basic abnormalities of cardiac rhythm. While there are limits to this tool, it does provide a framework with which you can approach the cardiac monitor while first learning to identify cardiac rhythms.

Cardiac arrest rhythms

Cardiac arrest occurs when a cardiac rhythm presents that is not capable of producing a cardiac output. There are four cardiac rhythms that are associated with cardiac arrest and you should be able to recognise each of these in an instant. They are:

- VT (broad complex tachycardia)
- VF
- Asystole
- EA.

Of these four rhythms, VT and VF are the most treatable by defibrillation and good-quality CPR. Asystole and PEA, however, have a poor prognosis unless a reversible cause can be found and promptly resolved.

Managing arrhythmias

The management of an arrhythmia in the acute setting will depend on a number of factors, the most important of which is how much of an impact that arrhythmia is having on the patient and, importantly, establishing if there are there any adverse signs present. Box 6.4 lists findings that indicate when immediate and aggressive management is required if the patient is to have the best possible of outcomes.

BOX 6.4 Findings in the presence of arrhythmia that command immediate management

- Systolic blood pressure <90 mmHg
- Heart rate <40 bpm
- Ventricular arrhythmias compromising blood pressure
- Recent asystole
- Second degree heart block type 2
- Complete heart block with broad QRS
- Ventricular pauses >3 seconds

(Continued)

(Continued)

- Reduced level of consciousness
- Chest pain
- Heart failure

The management of arrhythmias can be split into electrical and chemical interventions. Electrical interventions include defibrillation, cardioversion and the use of pacemakers. Chemical interventions involve the use of drugs that have an influence on the heart. The Resuscitation Council UK (2010) provides up-to-date protocols for the management of tachycardias with a pulse, bradycardia and cardiac arrest. These should form the basis of management.

The electrical management of arrhythmias serves either to add electrical stimulation to the heart or to remove excessive electrical activity from the heart. Defibrillation and cardioversion both seek to remove electrical activity in arrhythmias where there are either multiple pacemaker sites (such as in AF or VF) or a re-entry of the conducted electrical activity (which occurs in some narrow complex tachycardias). Both defibrillation and cardioversion work by exposing the heart to a massive amount of energy over a very short period of time. They are both used primarily in the management of tachycardias and uncoordinated rhythms such as VF. The intention is to simultaneously cause depolarisation of all the myocardium and conducting system cells, thus removing any additional electrical impulses in the heart and allowing the SA node to recover its rightful position as the pacemaker of the heart. Essentially, both defibrillation and cardioversion can be seen as treatments calling the heart to order. Defibrillation and cardioversion are delivered by the same piece of equipment, the only difference being that defibrillation occurs in the context of VF, where there is no pulse, and cardioversion occurs when the patient still has a pulse.

Defibrillation was once only performed by doctors, paramedics and specialist coronary care nurses. With the advent of automated external defibrillators (AEDs) more people can provide defibrillation. The use of an AED should be seen as an essential skill for all health professionals as shortening the time to defibrillation even by a few seconds dramatically improves outcomes. AEDs are simple to operate and training in their application can be provided in as little as three hours. The general procedure used in operating an AED is outlined in Box 6.5.

BOX 6.5 General procedure for the use of an automated external defibrillator

1 Verify cardiac arrest is present
2 Turn on the defibrillator
3 Apply pads to the patient's bare chest as illustrated on the pads. If the person is particularly hairy, rapid shaving using a safety razor may be required. The sternal pad is placed next to the sternum and below the clavicle on the right side of the chest. The apex pad is placed over the apex of the heart on the left lateral chest wall.
4 Follow the instructions given by the voice prompts of the defibrillator
5 If advised to administer a shock ensure all rescuers are stood clear of the patient before you do so
6 Continue to follow the voice prompts until help arrives

Cardioversion differs from defibrillation slightly in that the delivery of the shock is synchronised to the R wave of the QRS, thus preventing the delivery of the shock in the period of the cardiac cycle where there is a risk of creating VF. Cardioversion is used to treat rapid rhythms that are causing a haemodynamic compromise. Cardioversion in patients with a pulse must be performed under sedation.

Pacemakers are used to inject additional energy into the heart on an intermittent pulse-like basis in order to create a heart beat. Pacemakers are usually used to treat bradycardia and heart blocks. In emergencies, pacing can be transcutaneous (through the skin) where large adhesive pads are placed on the chest and an electrical current passes through them in order to stimulate the heart. Due to the resistance of the skin and lungs, a large amount of energy is needed and this is uncomfortable for the patient and thus can only be used in true emergencies in conscious patients. Again, sedation should be used when this is necessary. A more permanent solution is to use a pacing wire, which is inserted into the heart through a central venous catheter. This transvenous pacing uses less energy due to its proximity to the heart and is therefore more comfortable for the patient and more suited to longer-term temporary pacing. Later, the patient can be fitted with a permanent (implanted) pacemaker if this is deemed necessary. Figure 6.22 shows an ECG that is typical of a patient with a pacemaker in situ. Note the pacing spike in place of a P wave prior to the QRS complex.

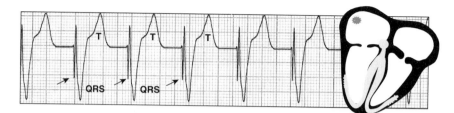

FIGURE 6.22   *Paced cardiac rhythm. Absence of P wave replaced by pacing spike (shown by arrow) prior to each QRS.*

Conclusion

ECG monitoring is an important tool in caring for the acutely ill as it provides additional information about the patient's health. The three-lead ECG is helpful in providing information about the heart rhythm. Other than this, it is limited in its usefulness and will require augmenting with 12-lead records. A basic understanding of the cardiac rhythms can be quickly gained. Being able to identify cardiac arrhythmias is an essential skill for those working with the acutely ill, as their presence often precedes cardiac arrest, and immediate recognition, coupled with aggressive intervention, can optimise the patient's outcome.

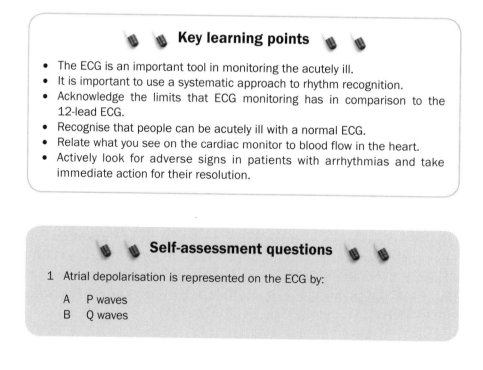

🔑 🔑 Key learning points 🔑 🔑

- The ECG is an important tool in monitoring the acutely ill.
- It is important to use a systematic approach to rhythm recognition.
- Acknowledge the limits that ECG monitoring has in comparison to the 12-lead ECG.
- Recognise that people can be acutely ill with a normal ECG.
- Relate what you see on the cardiac monitor to blood flow in the heart.
- Actively look for adverse signs in patients with arrhythmias and take immediate action for their resolution.

🔑 🔑 Self-assessment questions 🔑 🔑

1   Atrial depolarisation is represented on the ECG by:

   A   P waves
   B   Q waves

C   R waves
D   T waves
E   U waves

2 The normal cardiac cycle occurs within:

A   0.2 seconds
B   0.5 seconds
C   0.8 seconds
D   1.5 seconds
E   1.8 seconds

3 The resting state of myocardial cells is said to be:

A   Polarised
B   Depolarised
C   Repolarised
D   Charged
E   Ectopic

4 Normal cardiac rhythms originate from:

A   The Bundle of His
B   Atrioventricular node
C   Sinoatrial node
D   The left bundle branch
E   The Purkinje fibres

5 If there were multiple ectopic pacemaker sites in the ventricles, which
   rhythm would you expect to see on the ECG?

A   Atrial fibrillation
B   Ventricular fibrillation
C   Ventricular tachycardia
D   Ventricular ectopic
E   Unifocal premature ventricular contractions

6 Look at the rhythm strip shown below and identify the cardiac rhythm shown.

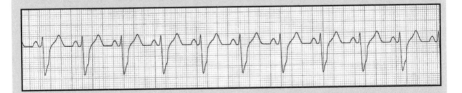

A   Atrial fibrillation
B   Sinus tachycardia
C   Normal sinus rhythm

(Continued)

(Continued)

    D   Sinus bradycardia
    E   Narrow complex tachycardia

7 Look at the rhythm strip shown below and identify the cardiac rhythm shown:

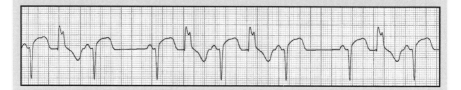

    A   Broad complex tachycardia
    B   First degree heart block
    C   Normal sinus rhythm
    D   Sinus bradycardia with premature ventricular contraction
    E   Ventricular tachycardia

8 Look at the rhythm strip shown below and identify the cardiac rhythm shown.

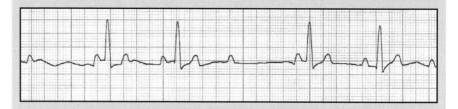

    A   First degree heart block
    B   Second degree heart block type 1
    C   Second degree heart block type 2
    D   Third degree heart block
    E   Complete heart block

9 Defibrillation seeks to restore normal cardiac rhythm by:

    A   Placing extra energy into the heart to replace lost ATP
    B   Depolarising all of the cardiac cells simultaneously, allowing order to be restored
    C   Forcing a sinoatrial impulse
    D   Speeding conduction down the Bundle of His
    E   Slowing conduction at the sinoatrial node

10 Pacemakers are most commonly used to treat:

A   Ventricular tachycardia
B   Bradycardias
C   Narrow complex tachycardia
D   Sinus tachycardia
E   Re-entrant tachycardias

Answers

1A, 2C, 3A, 4C, 5B, 6C, 7D, 8B, 9B, 10B.

Further reading

Hampton, J.R. (2003) *The ECG Made Easy*. London: Churchill Livingstone.
This is a popular text that expands on this chapter. It explains not only rhythm recognition but also facets of the 12-lead ECG.

Jenkins, R.D. and Gerred, S.J. (2005) *ECGs by Example*. London: Churchill Livingstone.
This book provides good quality examples of ECGs that can be used to practise ECG interpretation skills. Each ECG is accompanied by an explanation of its key findings.

National Collaborating Centre for Chronic Conditions. (2006) *Atrial Fibrillation: National Clinical Guideline for Management in Primary and Secondary Care*. London: Royal College of Physicians.
This guideline describes how atrial fibrillation should be managed in patients who present with this arrhythmia.

Nolan, J.P., Deakin, C.D., Soar, J., Bottiger, B.W. and Smith, G. (2005) 'European Resuscitation Council Guidelines for Resuscitation 2005, Section 4, Adult Advanced Life Support', *Resuscitation*, 67 (Suppl.): S1–S189.
This guideline outlines the management of the key arrhythmias that will be encountered in practice.

7

Responding to the acutely ill patient

Chapter aims

By the end of this chapter you should be able to:

- Describe an organised and systematic approach to those who are acutely ill
- Ensure that the care you give is goal directed
- Recognise the need to summon appropriate assistance and communicate the urgency of the situation correctly to colleagues

In the previous chapters specific aspects of the care of those who are acutely ill were described. While these chapters have provided vital underpinning knowledge they are limited in linking this information to the real-life scenarios that you are likely to encounter. Most often acutely ill patients present not with an isolated airway, breathing or circulation problem, but with a problem that causes widespread disruption in the body, requiring a range of supportive interventions from healthcare professionals. This chapter links the knowledge that you have gained in the previous chapters and aims to provide you with an organised approach that you can use to systematically assess and respond to the needs of those who have become acutely ill.

Basic rules of acute care

When responding to those who have been identified as being acutely ill there are some basic rules that you should adhere to. These rules will help to ensure that the care you give is focused on optimising the patient's condition. The rules that should be uppermost in your mind when you encounter a person who is acutely ill are summarised in Box 7.1.

BOX 7.1   Acute care rules

- Call for help early; never be afraid of calling for help
- Follow the ABCDE (airway, breathing, circulation, disability, exposure) model of care
- Treat any life-threatening problems as you find them
- Focus your efforts on keeping the person alive and not on trying to work out a definitive diagnosis
- Check to see that your interventions are working
- Continually reassess the patient; take nothing for granted

Call for help early; never be afraid of calling for help

All too often healthcare professionals delay calling for help when a patient is acutely ill. The reasons for this are various and are likely to include being unsure about how acutely ill a person is, not wanting to waste the time of others, not wanting to appear as if they have overreacted or cannot cope. Previous experiences of difficulty in obtaining help for an acutely ill person are also likely to have an impact on the behaviour of health professionals when considering decisions about calling for help.

Most acutely ill patients in hospital do not receive an appropriate or timely response and this has a negative impact on their likely survival. The acute care that is described in this book is designed to buy time until a more senior colleague can take over the care and provide definitive management for the patient's underlying condition. Remember it is better to explain to a doctor why you called for help than to explain to a coroner why you did not.

Follow the ABCDE model of care

The ABCDE model of care is explained later in this chapter. Following this model provides you with an organised framework that will ensure you address all of the points that are needed to keep a person alive.

Treat any life-threatening problems as you find them

As you progress through the ABCDE model of care, should you encounter anything which is life-threatening, stop and treat it, then continue with the remainder of your assessment. For example if you discover that a person has a blocked airway then you need to treat this before you should resolve a circulation problem.

Focus your efforts on keeping the person alive and not on trying to work out a definitive diagnosis

In the initial stages of managing the acutely ill person, it matters little what has caused the patient's problem. What matters more is that the person has a clear airway, that they are breathing and that their circulation is effective. Focusing your efforts on these essential aspects of care will help to keep the person alive until more definitive care can be given.

Check to see that your interventions are working

All of the interventions provided during the management of an acutely ill person are intended to achieve a specific aim. Performing a head tilt–chin lift, for example, is intended to open the airway. It is vital to ensure that if you perform an intervention, you check to see if it has worked. If your intervention fails to provide the expected outcome then you will need to do something more to achieve your aim. Keep at the back of your mind 'Why am I doing this and has it worked?'

Continually reassess the patient; take nothing for granted

In patients who are acutely ill their condition can change rapidly – a patient who had a pulse a short while earlier can soon lose it. The people caring for an acutely ill person can easily become distracted while trying to assist in another aspect of the patient's care and may start to neglect the task that they were already performing. Continually ensure that the patient is getting the care that you think they need. Check that the airway remains clear, that the oxygen has not become disconnected and intravenous lines have not infiltrated.

The ABCDE model of care

The ABCDE of resuscitation (Box 7.2) is something that all healthcare professionals are likely to have encountered either in their initial training or following on from it. It is, however, likely that resuscitation is where you have left the ABCDE model. The ABCDE approach has much to contribute to the recognition and care of the acutely ill, as it forces you to assess and treat the important physiological domains that malfunction during episodes of acute illness. While most professionals have at least heard of 'airway, breathing, circulation', significantly fewer professionals have come across the 'D' (disability) and 'E' (exposure) aspects of this model. Disability relates mainly to brain and nervous system function, and exposure relates to the removal of all clothes so that a head-to-toe examination can be undertaken in order to identify anything that has gone unnoticed, such as a wound infection in a patient with a septic picture or a per rectal blood loss in a patient with a low blood pressure.

BOX 7.2   The ABCDE model

- A – Airway
- B – Breathing
- C – Circulation
- D – Disability
- E – Exposure

The proliferation of the ABCDE model as one that is useful in the assessment of all acutely ill patients may have been hampered in the past by the way in which it was taught (Kaye et al., 1991; Leah and Coats, 1999). In many resuscitation classes where the ABCDE is mostly discussed, answers to questions such as 'Is the airway intact?', 'Is the person breathing normally?' and 'Are there signs of circulation?' are largely yes or no answers. In patients who are so acutely ill that they have suffered a cardiac arrest, these responses are wholly appropriate, yet in patients who have not yet deteriorated to cardiac arrest the ABCDE model still holds tremendous worth. The questions that must be asked though are more diverse and form a part of a deductive information-gathering process. Modern resuscitation and acute care courses now acknowledge this point and have built on the ABCDE approach, showing its wider relevance to all acutely ill patients (Smith et al., 2002; Soar et al., 2003; Berry and Stevens, 2008).

Applying the ABCDE approach to the acutely ill

The international resuscitation community has done much to support the advancement of the ABCDE approach to the acutely ill patient prior to the onset of cardiac arrest (Nolan and Baskett, 2005; Resuscitation Council UK, 2005; International Liaison Committee on Resuscitation, 2010). The following represents a summary of the most important parts of these guidelines for use in the initial stages of caring for the acutely ill patient while awaiting the arrival of more experienced help.

When you encounter an acutely ill person your first priority is to summon help. Exactly how you do this will depend on the location that you are working in, your level of training and the clinical urgency of the situation. Summoning help in a clinical setting will often be a two-stage approach that involves shouting for immediate assistance and then telephoning for help. Ensuring that help is on the way early will reduce any delays to definitive care. The intention of shouting for help is to enlist people working in the local environment to assist you in responding to the patient's needs. When you shout for help be clear about what the problem is and what assistance you require. Do not be ambiguous. Statements such as 'Can I get a hand here please?' are not specific and they do not communicate urgency; if staff are committed elsewhere they may ignore or delay responding to your request. Be very specific in requests for help by saying something like 'Help! cardiac arrest! Call the crash team, bring the emergency trolley to bay two.' Co-workers in your area should be trained to respond to such requests for assistance by shouting back to confirm that help is on its way.

The next stage is to try to elicit a response from the patient to assess their level of consciousness. Ask the patient loudly 'Are you all right?' If there is no response, shake the person's shoulders and ask them again 'Are you all right?' Use the AVPU scale (Chapter 3) to quantify the person's responsiveness. If they provide an orientated verbal response then, for the time being, they have a clear airway and are conscious. If they only respond to shaking, or they are unconscious, then the airway is at risk and you must consider this.

Your next priority is to open the airway using a head tilt–chin lift manoeuvre if there is no risk of cervical spinal injury. If there is a risk of cervical spinal injury then the jaw thrust manoeuvre may be safer. Look in the mouth to see if there is any debris or fluid present. Suction any fluid out of the person's mouth, using a Yankauer sucker, suctioning only what you can see. Be careful not to invoke the gag reflex while suctioning as this may provoke vomiting. If the patient is vomiting, roll them on to their side to allow the vomit to drain from the mouth. Remove any broken or poorly fitting dentures but leave well-fitting dentures in place.

With the airway held open, assess the person's breathing. Place your cheek next to the person's mouth and nose. You should be looking towards the patient's feet. From this position you will be able to feel any air movement on your cheek, hear any breath sounds and see any movement of the chest. Decide if the person is breathing normally or not breathing normally. Take no longer than ten seconds to do this. Breathing normally means that the person is moving air at an acceptable rate. Not breathing normally may mean that the person:

- Has stopped breathing
- Is taking occasional gasps
- Is breathing too slowly or too rapidly.

If the person has stopped breathing, or is only taking occasional gasps, it is likely that the person's heart has stopped beating and they have experienced a cardiac arrest. Look for signs of life such as movement or coughing. If you are experienced in assessing carotid pulses you may feel for a carotid pulse, although research shows that most health professionals are not able to reliably determine the presence or absence of a carotid pulse during emergencies (Eberle et al., 1996; Moule, 2000; Tibballs and Russell, 2009). Take no longer than ten seconds to assess for signs of life. If there are no signs of life and/or no carotid pulse can be felt, or there is doubt over whether a carotid pulse is present or absent, then you should start cardiopulmonary resuscitation (CPR). Attach the person to the defibrillator and attempt defibrillation if you are trained to do so and it is clinically indicated. Then alternate two minutes of CPR with defibrillation attempts until the resuscitation team arrives. When the team arrives hand over to them, explain what has happened and the treatment that you have given; do not stop the CPR until someone takes over from you. If there are sufficient staff available then you should attempt to insert an intermediate airways device, such as a laryngeal mask airway, and ventilate the person through this while awaiting the arrival of the resuscitation team.

If the person is breathing and shows signs of life then continue to support the airway. Decide if the person needs any support with the airway such as an oropharyngeal airway or an intermediate airway device. Administer oxygen to the person via a non-rebreathe mask or a self-inflating bag with an oxygen reservoir if an intermediate airway device is in place. Next, attach the monitoring equipment to the person as a minimum – this should include pulse oximetry, non-invasive blood pressure measuring and electrocardiograph. If the respiratory rate is fewer than 8 or more than 30 per minute consider supporting the person's breathing with either a pocket mask or a self-inflating bag. Establish intravenous access if not already present and draw blood at the same time for a full blood count and urea and electrolytes as a minimum. Then use your knowledge of breathing and circulation problems to identify if there are any immediate life-threatening problems present and provide the treatment that you are authorised to give. Think specifically about a need to give a fluid challenge in order to bolster circulation. Then check the person's blood glucose level and perform a head-to-toe examination to check for any clues as to the cause of their condition. Only perform these actions if they will not interrupt care of the airway, breathing and circulation. Then reassess everything and start to consider specific causes for the patient's condition.

Telephoning for help

Responding to the needs of the acutely ill is a multiprofessional effort and help will need to be summoned from an appropriate source. The first step when it comes to obtaining help is to decide what type of response the person you are caring for requires if their needs are to be met most effectively. This will be governed by the extent to which the person has deteriorated and the options for response that are available in your work setting. In some small community hospitals or in primary care the best response may well be a 999 call to the ambulance service. In a larger, more acute hospital setting the options available are likely to be more diverse.

For patients who have experienced a cardiac or respiratory arrest, the crash or resuscitation team should be called out. In England there is now a standard telephone number in hospitals, '2222', which can be dialled to activate the members of a resuscitation team. Increasingly, with recognition of the poor outcomes following an episode of acute illness, many hospitals are now developing medical emergency teams (MET) or critical care outreach teams (CCOTs). These are often multidisciplinary teams that can be called when a patient experiences a physiological decline, but has not yet had a cardiac or respiratory arrest. In some centres the MET and crash teams function as one. In hospitals that do not have a MET or a CCOT and you come across a patient who has a significant deterioration in their condition, do not be afraid to call the resuscitation team.

Information that you communicate will depend on the clinical urgency of the situation and to whom you are talking. If the patient has had a cardiac arrest, it is sufficient to tell the operator 'cardiac arrest, ward two' and then get the operator to repeat it back to you so that you know they have heard you correctly. In this situation you need to communicate the clinical problem and the exact location in which you require help. If, however, you are talking to a doctor you may need to provide additional information. Many people have reported difficulties in enlisting help from medical staff for a patient who they believe to be unwell. The reasons for this are likely to be many, but there are things that can be done to ensure good working relationships and an appropriate response for the patient. When communicating with a clinician, it is essential to be clear about:

- Who and where you are
- What is wrong
- How urgent the situation is
- What you want the person to do.

Then agree an action plan.

Phrases such as, 'I have a feeling this lady is not well' or 'When you have a second' or 'He is just not right' do little to communicate either the urgency or severity of the situation and the person to whom you are speaking may prioritise other patients who may well be more stable than your patient, but who received a better representation of their case. Telling the person the vital signs (minimum dataset) and the early warning score helps to communicate both the urgency and severity of the situation. See Box 7.3 for an example conversation between a nurse and a doctor.

BOX 7.3   Example conversation to enlist medical help

Who and where you are:
Hello Dr Taylor, its Caroline Palmer, Staff Nurse on Ward 10 here.

What is wrong:
I have a 65-year-old woman admitted this morning with pneumonia. Obs now are RR 30, Pulse 115 and irregular, BP 95/62. Previously alert now responding only to voice. Her SaO_2 is 89% despite 60% oxygen.

(Continued)

(Continued)

How urgent the situation is:
This is a sudden deterioration in her condition from her last assessment, where all observations were normal.

What you want the person to do:
Please can you come to ward 10 immediately to see her?

Then decide on an action plan:
Thanks Caroline, I will come immediately. Can you give her 15L of oxygen via a non-rebreathe mask. Ensure that she has intravenous access and record an ECG while I make my way to the ward.

No problem, Clive. So that's 15L of oxygen via a non-rebreathe mask; ensure that she has intravenous access and record a 12-lead ECG. I shall do that now.

Thanks, see you on Ward 10 shortly.

If you experience difficulty in enlisting help then you must make clear your concerns about this patient and the urgency of the situation. If after repeated attempts at communicating the scenario, you are still unable to secure assistance you should make clear to the doctor that you intend to seek help elsewhere. A way of doing this initially might be to ask the doctor if they can suggest from where you might be able to enlist help with this patient. Remember, you remain accountable and it is your duty to seek help (Health Professions Council, 2008; Nursing and Midwifery Council, 2008). If the first doctor refuses to attend the patient and you remain concerned, then you must seek help from another source or you could be held negligent for failing to securing appropriate help for the patient.

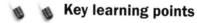

Key learning points

- Constantly ask yourself – do you need help? And call for it early.
- Be confident when asking for help. Communicate the urgency of the situation and what you want the person to do.
- Use the ABCDE model to respond to the acutely ill.
- Treat all life-threatening problems as you find them.
- Ensure that your interventions are working. If not do something more.

Self-assessment questions

1   If you are concerned about an acutely ill person and are unable to secure medical help despite explaining the assessments you have undertaken and stressing the urgency, you should:

A   Document this and reassess the patient later
B   Call the resuscitation team
C   Inform the doctor of your ongoing concerns and seek help from another source
D   Proceed to treat the person as you see fit without medical involvement
E   Ask a nurse to confirm your assessment

2   The standardised telephone number to summon the resuscitation team in hospitals in England is:

A   3333
B   2222
C   5555
D   2999
C   999

3   The intention of exposing the patient is to:

A   Cool them
B   Provide access in case emergency surgery becomes necessary
C   Allow the monitoring attachments to be placed
D   Enable examination of the patient
E   Make the person more comfortable

4   Which of the following would indicate that CPR was needed?

A   A palpable carotid pulse
B   Rapid breathing
C   Absence of normal breathing and no movements
D   Slow breathing (8 breaths per minute)
E   Absence of a radial pulse with a palpable carotid

5   If you discover your patient has a life-threatening problem you should:

A   Carry on and complete a full A–E assessment
B   Ask colleague to confirm the problem
C   Stop further assessments, shout for help and treat the patient's problem
D   Insert an intermediate airway device
E   Start CPR

Answers

1C, 2B, 3D, 4C, 5C.

Further reading

Adam, S. and Osborne, S. (2005) *Critical Care Nursing Science and Practice*. Oxford: Oxford University Press.
This text provides details about the type of care that a person who is acutely ill can expect to receive in the critical care unit. It provides a good insight into this area of practice.

Harrison, R. and Daly, L. (2006) *Acute Medical Emergencies: A Nursing Guide*. Edinburgh: Churchill Livingstone.
This is a handy pocket-sized text that presents more detail on the specific medical emergencies that are commonly encountered in practice.

8

Significant others, breaking bad news

Chapter aims

By the end of this chapter you should be able to:

- Explain the importance of significant others in the care of people who are acutely ill
- Prepare for circumstances where there is a need to break bad news
- Describe methods of breaking bad news
- Predict the possible reactions that people may display on hearing bad news
- Provide initial support and arrange continuing support for people after learning of a loved one's illness or death

Breaking the bad news of a person's sudden illness or death to a relative, friend or partner is a tremendous responsibility and one that needs to be taken seriously. There is much potential for health professionals to cause additional stress and long-standing emotional upset if the situation is not carefully managed. All too often, though, health professionals receive poor quality of preparation for this critical duty and are often unsure of how to go about breaking bad news and supporting loved ones optimally.

Like technical clinical skills, being able to engage with a person at a time of loss and assist them through their emotions requires a theoretical back-drop and practice. A caring, empathic and sensitive health professional can go a great way to securing an effective, trusting relationship with significant others, for which they will undoubtedly be thankful in the future.

Insensitivity and arrogance, however, will damage the relationship, be long remembered and discussed with many different people.

While there are no universally accepted rules or standards for breaking bad news and supporting people at a time of loss, there exists a body of knowledge that highlights the value of some key principles that should be present when dealing with people at times of loss. This chapter will provide an overview of the key issues that health professionals should consider when undertaking this vital aspect of their role.

The importance of people

Many reading this book will have experienced the loss of a loved one or someone close. For those who to have not experienced this, the threat of losing someone is bad enough. What is clear is that people are all-important and that we need people around us to provide love and support. As health professionals, we must recognise that this is a two-way process – the patients in our care will need the support of those close to them; their significant others will often need support themselves in managing the emotions that are triggered by seeing a person close to them extremely ill or dying, or who has been recently bereaved. An essential aspect of the health professional's role is to recognise the significance of people and facilitate a process of support that is appropriate in meeting everyone's needs.

Society is now tremendously diverse and people live in a wide range of relationships different from those that would have traditionally been recognised. For some, traditional relationships will exist, but increasingly for others there may be same-sex relationships, civil partnerships or simply close friends who provide the bulk of a person's social and emotional support. These relationships must be recognised and given equal worth as would have been shown to a more traditional relationship, as the emotional upset that is experienced is identical. Due to the variety of relationships that exist in contemporary society, the term 'significant others' has been coined to describe those whom the patient identifies as being significant to them. Failing to respect this can cause extreme distress on both sides and complicate a person's grieving.

An approach to breaking bad news

The process of breaking bad news is one that starts long before a person becomes sick or injured. The starting point is to ensure that there is an appropriate infrastructure in place to allow bad news to be broken in the optimal manner when the need arises. To aid in the process of breaking bad news it is perhaps helpful to split the topic into the phases of:

- Preparation
- Summoning the significant others
- Preparing the significant others
- Breaking the bad news
- Supporting people after the death of a significant other

Preparation

Preparation for breaking bad news involves both personal preparation and environmental preparation. Personal preparation will involve any training that you may need before attempting to break bad news to a person as well as preparing yourself mentally for what you are about to do. As a part of personal preparation, you may rehearse with a colleague or in your head what you will say to the significant others when they arrive.

Environmental preparation will involve ensuring that there is a suitable, private space where the news can be broken. Every hospital should have a relatives' room located close to the clinical area. This should be a comfortable room with sofas, drink-making facilities, tissues and a wash basin, as a minimum. It should be pleasantly decorated; fresh flowers are ideal. For practical reasons, the door should have a sign that states clearly when the room is in use, to avoid interruptions at key moments. Breaking bad news can provoke a strong emotional response which can manifest as aggression or as a medical problem, and for this reason the room should be equipped with a panic button. Having such an environment for breaking bad news will make the experience more tolerable for all involved as well as facilitating best practice in communication. If you need to break bad news you should check that the room is free, clean and suitably prepared.

Summoning the significant others

The first point to consider is who needs to be informed about the situation. While this may seem obvious when a patient has been in hospital for some time and the contact details are documented in the notes, there will be times when this is more complex, for example when the identities of those significant to the patient are not known. In some circumstances, for instance where a person has been admitted unconscious or with significant cognitive deficit, there may difficulties in contacting the significant others. The 'ICE' campaign started by paramedic Bob Brotchie encourages people to store the details of who they would like to be informed 'in case of emergency' under the name of 'ICE' in their mobile phone, and this may help in some circumstances (BBC, 2005). Where this is not the case mobile phones can still be used for information as can other personal effects that the patient may have with them.

Once those who are to be informed have been identified, the next consideration is locating them and positively confirming their relationship with the patient. Find out if the relatives are in the hospital or if they need to be summoned to the hospital. If the relatives are already in the hospital, then they should be taken to the relatives' room so that they can be kept up to date with changes as they occur. If the relatives are not in the hospital then they should be contacted by telephone and asked to attend the hospital. The following points should be included in the telephone conversation when asking a relative to come to the hospital:

- Who you are
- Who the patient is
- What has happened to them (in brief, e.g. car accident, sudden illness)
- That the condition is serious
- Can they come to the hospital (name and location)?
- Where in the hospital they should go
- Not to rush or drive in a distressed state.

If it is not possible to contact people via telephone, the local constabulary will normally assist in breaking the news of an accident, injury or sudden illness. Often the police may also be able to help with transport to the hospital in such circumstances.

Preparing the significant others

When relatives arrive at the hospital, they should be met promptly and not made to feel uncomfortable. Personnel who are likely to encounter the person first, such as reception staff, should be made aware of the person's impending arrival so that they can accommodate them without delay, quickly making the clinical team aware of their arrival. People who have been informed that someone whom they love has become critically ill are likely to be extremely anxious. This should be anticipated and strategies put in place to mitigate and not escalate this.

While no death is easy to cope with, the predictability of the death can assist people in their response to grieving. If death occurs at the end of a period of illness it allows people time to start the mental preparation that is needed, while in a sudden death after an acute illness or injury no such opportunity is afforded. Where the patient and significant others are known to the health professionals and a relationship has developed, it may be easier to break the news of a death. That said, however, news of an expected death should not be considered to cause less distress to those significant to the patient. Deaths that occur suddenly are associated with a poorer response to grieving. This is probably the case as there is a lack of opportunity for mental preparation. When death is a possibility, health professionals should employ strategies that help people to prepare for the possibility that their loved one may die. It is often possible to provide an accelerated mental preparation of people for the news that they may ultimately hear.

One of the best ways to prepare people for the news of a potential death is to be open and honest, keeping them informed of developments as they occur. It is crucial not to give false hope if a situation is serious and there is potential for death to occur. Phrases that convey the severity of the situation in simple language are needed. An example is 'Mr Abbot's condition is serious. We are actively treating him, but we need to see how he responds to treatment before I can tell you any more about the likely outcome.' This is both honest and conveys the uncertainty of the situation. If cardiac arrest has occurred then relatives should be made aware of this in an understandable manner as death is a real risk here and the significant others should be aware of this possibility: 'I have just been with Mr Abbot. At the moment he is not breathing and his heart is not beating. The medical team are working to restart his heart, but the situation is very grave and there is a chance that he may die soon.' Pause and respond to questions, and then ask: 'Would you like to be with Mr Abbott while the medical team are treating him?'

In the past, those significant to the patient were often whisked away quickly at the mere thought that a resuscitation might become necessary. More recently resuscitations witnessed by significant others have been demonstrated to be something that can assist people in recognising the seriousness of the situation and enable them to see that everything that could be done was done. This witnessed resuscitation can assist in accelerating the mental preparation needed to make sense of the news of a death if this will need to be given later.

To facilitate witnessed resuscitation, someone, usually a nurse, should explain in understandable terms what is likely to be seen before the significant other enters the resuscitation area. They should be told that they can leave at any time if they are distressed by what they see. Opportunities should be found to allow the person to hold the patient's hand and talk to them, but the person must be told of the need to let go when asked, so as not to delay treatments such as defibrillation. The same nurse should stay with the significant other and explain again in simple terms each procedure that is performed and how it will help the person. Many people are thankful to be with their loved one at this time and gain great reassurance from being with them at the end of their life. Staff fears about having people witness resuscitation should not be allowed to deny people this important opportunity. On a practical note, it is important to ensure that the resuscitation is being competently and professionally performed before inviting the significant others to witness it.

Where significant others are present during resuscitation, it may be necessary to break the news of the death in the resuscitation area. The team leader should approach the person, introduce themselves and explain the condition, treatment given and the position that has been reached. Resuscitation should continue while this discussion is taking place until the team leader gives a signal to stop the resuscitation. At no point should the significant other be asked if they want the resuscitation to stop as this shifts the responsibility for decision making onto them. Such a request could complicate their grieving with thoughts like 'If only I had said to carry on maybe they would have survived.' A decision to stop an established resuscitation is a medical decision and requires medical knowledge that is not available to lay people. Significant others should not be expected to make such a decision without the benefit of such information.

Breaking the bad news

While there is no totally right or wrong way of breaking bad news, there are things that can be done to make the process easier for all involved. It is necessary to remember that each situation is unique and you will need to adapt your technique to be optimally effective while incorporating the basic principles of good practice. In particular, there is a need to be respectful and culturally competent in your approach. Where English is not the person's first language, a suitable interpreter should be sought. Every effort should be made not to use relatives as interpreters, as they themselves are likely to be distressed and it is impossible to assess the information that they will pass on or withhold.

Who should break bad news will depend on whether the death is sudden or expected and the sort of relationships that have been forged, and indeed the circumstances that have arisen. After a sudden death, the most senior doctor who has been caring for the patient is the ideal choice of person, but if there is a delay in contacting this team member or they are not available, the duty may fall to a nurse who has knowledge of the case. If the death is expected then the nurse with whom the significant others have developed a relationship is the ideal choice. It is important to check whether there are any local protocols that need to be adhered to, as well as considering the legal, ethical and professional issues that relate to information sharing and breaching of confidentiality (Caldicott, 1997; Health Professions Council, 2008; HM Government, 2008; Nursing and Midwifery Council, 2008).

When it comes to the act of breaking bad news, it is important to consider what you say and how you say it. Prepare yourself for the task of breaking bad news by changing any blood-stained clothing and ensuring that you are smart and presentable. Think about what you are going to say. Make sure that colleagues know what you are about to do, so that they do not come looking for you and interrupt at a critical time. Take someone with you who can help to support you and the relatives. The following points should then feature in all conversations where bad news needs to be broken.

- Introduce yourself to the relatives. Give your name and explain your role.
- Identify who you are talking to and check that you have the right relatives for the right patient (never neglect this).
- Identify who is the principal significant other.
- Get on the same level of the person, ideally sitting.
- Check what the relatives know has happened so far.
- Explain briefly and in lay terms what has happened and the treatment given.
- Where applicable, say that the person has died; do not use euphemisms like 'passed on' or 'gone upstairs'.
- Give the people time to react.
- Offer an opportunity to ask questions and check the person's understanding.
- Allow the relatives time to view the person. Use the patient's name. Do not use terms such as 'the body'.
- Let the relatives be alone with the person.

Box 8.1 details an example conversation between a health professional and a patient's relative.

BOX 8.1   Example conversation in which bad news is broken

Health professional: Hello, my name is Sharon Harvey and I am one of the nurses who has been caring for Mr Abbott. I called you earlier today. Can I just check that you are the relatives of Mr James Abbott?

Significant other: Yes. I am his wife and this is our daughter Andrea.

Health professional: I have asked you come to the hospital because earlier today Mr Abbott developed some chest pain. Both a doctor and I saw him and he was diagnosed with having a heart attack and treatment was started for this. Shortly afterwards while I was with him his heart stopped beating. We started resuscitation and the other doctors arrived very quickly. We placed a breathing tube in his mouth and used electricity and drugs to stimulate his heart. His heart attack was severe. We used all the treatments possible, but I am afraid he did not respond to the treatment and Mr Abbot died a short while ago.

[Pause and respond to any questions or emotions]

[If you are unsure that the person has understood then it may be helpful to check their level of understanding. A simple question, such as the one below, can help you with this]

Do you understand what I have said to you both; is there anything that you would like to ask me?

[Pause and respond to any questions or emotions]

Would you like to see Mr Abbot now?

Significant others: Yes, please.

Health professional: I can arrange that. You need to know that he will still have the breathing tube in his mouth and a tube in his neck. We are not allowed to remove these yet so you need to prepare yourselves for that. I will go and check if it is okay to go in now. Please wait here a moment. I won't be long.

[Escort the significant others to the bedside and allow time to be alone with Mr Abbott. Go back after a short while and ensure that they are coping.

After viewing the deceased, take the significant others back to the relatives' room. Offer them a drink and answer any questions they may have. Offer to call anyone for support. Finally, explain the procedures that they must follow and offer them a *What to Do After Death* leaflet.]

If the relatives are not available to attend the hospital, it may be necessary to break bad news over the telephone. Breaking bad news over the telephone is highly undesirable for a range of reasons, although occasionally it may be necessary if the significant other is a great distance away and cannot get to the hospital. Where it does become necessary, the above points should be followed as far as possible. You should also attempt to assess the amount of support that a person may have close to them before breaking the news.

Supporting people after the death of a significant other

Reactions to the news that a significant other has died can be very varied, ranging from the initially dramatic, to the delayed and denied. Elisabeth Kübler-Ross (1973) identified five stages of grief that people commonly pass through when they encounter loss. While not all people will pass through these in the same way, or to the same degree, or in the same order, they represent some notable feelings that people can experience. The stages of grief are:

1 **Denial**: There is a feeling of disbelief that the death has occurred and there is a wish to carry on as normal.
2 **Anger**: This may be directed at themselves ('If only I had'); the person who has died ('How could you have been so stupid'); the medical team ('You're incompetent. I am going to sue you'); or some other person such as a driver in a road traffic collision. People can become furious that the death has taken place, even if, realistically, nothing could have stopped it. It is important to recognise that anger at this stage is a normal part of the grieving process and you should not resent the person for it. That said, neither should individuals who are grieving be allowed to threaten the safety of another person.
3 **Bargaining**: The person may have thoughts of 'If only it was me' or 'I would do anything to change the situation.'
4 **Depression**: The person may feel numb, although anger and sadness may remain underneath. They may experience thoughts of self-harm and, if this is the case, appropriate care should be provided as dictated by local protocols. Risk factors for a poor outcome of grieving are listed in Box 8.2.
5 **Acceptance**: This may take some time. Acceptance occurs where the anger, sadness and mourning have tapered off and the person accepts the reality of the loss and starts to return to normal functioning.

BOX 8.2 Risk factors for poor outcome following bereavement

Predisposing factors

- Ambivalent or dependent relationship
- Multiple prior bereavements

(Continued)

(Continued)

- Previous mental illness, especially depression
- Low self-esteem of bereaved person

Around the time of the death

- Sudden and unexpected death
- Untimely death of a younger person
- Preparation for their death
- Stigmatised deaths – HIV-related, suicide
- Culpable deaths
- Sex of bereaved person – elderly male widower, for example
- Caring for the deceased person more than six months
- Inability to carry out valued religious rituals

After the death

- Level of perceived social support
- Lack of opportunities for new interests
- Stress from other life crises

Source: Sheldon (2000)

Understanding the stages of grieving allows you to appreciate how the person may feel, and to provide them with reassurance that their feelings are quite normal. Touch, such as holding a person's hand or giving them a hug may be appropriate in some circumstances, although in other circumstances it will be wholly inappropriate. The culture of the person may dictate the appropriateness and there may be gender issues that need to be taken into consideration. Each clinician needs to read the situation and decide on an appropriate course of action. However, as a general rule if the person shows that they don't want to be touched then this must be respected.

It is important that social support is sought for the person. Initially, this may come from a nurse, but offers should be made to summon relatives or friends who can provide a personal slant and ongoing support. Religious support from the hospital chaplaincy may also be valued by some individuals. Most hospitals also have a social work service and these should be offered as a source of support to the recently bereaved.

Dealing with the administration of a death can be difficult as one tries not only to cope with the loss, but also to register the death and arrange a funeral. If this is a person's first experience of death they may not even know how to go about this or what indeed needs to be done. Written information such as the Department for Work and Pensions leaflet *What to do After a Death in England and Wales* is available and can give practical instructions.

To assist in achieving closure, a telephone call made to the significant other after a few days following the death, by a person who was involved in the patient care, can be a source of tremendous support to the bereaved individual. It provides an opportunity to ask any unanswered questions and shows that they are still in the thoughts of hospital staff.

Final considerations

Patient confidentiality should not be forgotten, as breaching this can have complex and far-reaching consequences for the patient both during the time of illness and in recovery. For the significant other, breaches of confidentiality can alter their memory of a patient and therefore caution needs to be exercised. Details that may seem insignificant, such as the location of a person's collapse prior to admission to hospital, can be incriminating and reveal information that could distress all parties. Likewise assumptions about what the patient has told significant others about their illness should not be made, as, again, this can reveal information that the patient might not have wanted to share.

In many deaths, there is an opportunity for the person to become an organ donor. Organ donation can give loved ones some sense of utility at a time of loss. Most hospitals have local guidelines on this issue and you should ensure that you are familiar with them and incorporate them into your practice as appropriate.

Depending on the circumstances of the death, permission may need to be sought for an autopsy examination. Seeking this permission can cause distress to the relatives, for obvious reasons. It is important to reassure the family that an autopsy is a medical procedure that is carried out by a doctor and that it will be conducted with respect for the person. Making a request for an autopsy examination or informing the significant others that a coroner's autopsy is required should be left to the doctor in charge of the patient's case.

Your feelings

Supporting the significant others of a person who is seriously ill or who has died can be tremendously difficult for health professionals, particularly if the situation is similar to one they have found themselves in at some time. Showing your emotions to significant others is a matter of some debate and requires a degree of assessment as to whether or not this is appropriate. Showing emotion can help to demonstrate empathy and illustrate that they are not just another case, and thus showing a tear can be appropriate. Conversely, it is important that the emotion shown is proportionate and does not detract from the goal of supporting the person through their experience. The demonstration of too much or uncontrolled emotion in front of the significant others could result in them feeling that their experience was devalued as their grief is likely to evoke stronger feelings than your own. A situation where the significant others end up consoling the health professional is unacceptable. Health professionals need to find ways of dealing with these feelings without bottling them up. Talking to a colleague about how you are feeling can be an important release and one that you should not be ashamed of using.

Conclusion

Breaking bad news is never an easy task to perform. The news that you have to impart will change a person's life forever. While there is no strictly right or wrong way of breaking bad news, there are some things that can be done to assist people to understand the information that is to be imparted and to start the process of grieving. People will remember for the rest of their lives the moment that they heard a person who was dear to them had died. There is no second chance at getting it right, so thought and planning must underpin any occasion when you are called on to break bad news. Being compassionate and empathetic will assist in the task of breaking bad news. Showing respect and honesty will assist a person with grieving.

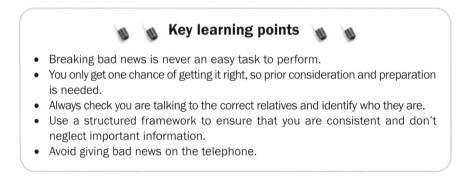

🔥 🔥 Key learning points 🔥 🔥

- Breaking bad news is never an easy task to perform.
- You only get one chance of getting it right, so prior consideration and preparation is needed.
- Always check you are talking to the correct relatives and identify who they are.
- Use a structured framework to ensure that you are consistent and don't neglect important information.
- Avoid giving bad news on the telephone.

- Be aware of the potential reactions to bad news.
- Do not assume that information has been taken in, and be prepared to repeat information several times.
- Allow the person to see the deceased after death, preparing them for the presence of intravenous lines or tracheal tubes.
- Do all you can to be empathetic and supportive.
- People should be enabled to undertake valued religious procedures.
- Ensure continued access to help.
- Make sure significant others are supported with administration after the death.
- Acknowledge your own feelings and talk about these with a colleague.

Self-assessment exercise

Reflect upon a time when you were required to break bad news or you witnessed bad news being broken. Write a list of the things that you thought were well handled on that occasion and those things that you think could have been improved. Next, do the same from the relative's point of view. Do you think that there are any differences?

Then write five action points that detail how you will improve your own practice when it comes to breaking bad news to people.

Further reading

Diamond, J. (2004) *C: Because Cowards Get Cancer Too*. London: Random House. While not an academic text, this book provides a thoughtful insight into one family's experience of receiving bad news on repeated occasions. It is both humorous and some may say challenging to traditional thinking in how bad news is broken.

Moss, B. (2008) *Communication Skills for Health & Social Care*. London: Sage Publications. This book provides an overview of communication skills needed for professional and engaging interactions.

Steane, A. (2007) *Who Cares? One Family's Shocking Story of Care in Today's NHS*. Bournemouth: Original Book.
This is a book that tells a story of how repeated failures to provide good-quality acute care impact on a family. The author explains how simple failures and the attitudes of hospital staff caused an amazing amount of distress. This is an essential read for those involved in delivering care to patients.

9

Legal, ethical and professional issues

Chapter aims

By the end of this chapter you should be able to:

- Describe the common legal, ethical and professional issues that can arise while caring for the acutely ill
- Identify circumstances where escalating care may not be in the best interests of patients
- Explain the role of decisions to withhold or withdraw life-prolonging medical treatment
- Contribute to decisions that involve withholding or withdrawing life-sustaining treatments

The practice of caring for the acutely ill and performing resuscitation is fraught with legal, professional and ethical issues. In emergency situations, life is often at stake and the atmosphere emotionally charged. As a result of the high potential for loss, many people have highly polarised views about what is the right thing to do in a given situation. While this is true for health professionals, patients and those who are significant to them are also likely to have strong views about what should happen and these must never be ignored. This chapter will explain how you can negotiate some of the difficult legal, professional and ethical issues that can be encountered in practice, with specific regard to caring for those who are acutely ill. While this chapter will not be able to provide guidance for each and every dilemma that you might encounter in practice, it intends, like the rest of this book to suggest guiding principles that can be used to inform thinking and practice.

Identifying legal, ethical and professional issues

There are many legal, ethical and professional (LEP) issues that influence the delivery of healthcare in general. The particular LEP issues that impact on the delivery of care to those who are acutely ill are part of this wider framework. The differences are such that when caring for a person who has become acutely ill, the LEP issues are often very obvious and the consequences of decisions made are irreversible and may lead to or involve a person's death. Some of the LEP issues that are pertinent to the care of those who are acutely ill are outlined in Box 9.1.

BOX 9.1 Legal, ethical and professional issues that impact on the care of those who are acutely ill

- Professional accountability
- Patient safety
- Negligence
- Withholding and withdrawing life-prolonging medical treatment
- Equality and diversity
- Record keeping
- Consent
- Confidentiality and data protection
- Health and safety

It is not within the scope of this chapter to address each and every one of the LEP issues in depth. The focus of this chapter will be the LEP knowledge needed to understand the issues that surround the withholding and withdrawing of life-prolonging medical treatment, which is a fundamental issue that arises frequently when the need for acute care is being considered.

Withholding and withdrawing life-prolonging medical treatment

Despite major advances in medical technologies and nursing care, healthcare is not able to cure all ills and there comes a time where illness or injury is too severe and death is an inevitable certainty. In these circumstances, the application of continued curative medical treatment is medically inappropriate as it serves no beneficial outcome for the patient. In fact, continuing to struggle in a medically hopeless case may be ethically deplorable as the intention of doing good cannot be realised and any artificial prolongation of life may lead to increased suffering, a loss of dignity and ultimately increased harm. The application of this principle in practice requires decisions about when a person has reached this point in life, the medical interventions that remain appropriate and those that have become inappropriate.

To do this successfully it is necessary to identify what constitutes life-prolonging treatment. The British Medical Association (BMA) (2007) defines life-prolonging treatment as 'all treatments or procedures that have the potential to postpone the patient's death'. Examples that the BMA offers include:

- Cardiopulmonary resuscitation (CPR)
- Artificial ventilation
- Curative chemotherapy
- Dialysis
- Antibiotics when given for potentially life-threatening infections
- Artificial nutrition and hydration.

Probably one of the most contentious of decisions a health professional will face is deciding who should receive treatment and for whom continued curative treatment has become inappropriate and should be withheld. Indeed, this topic has been the subject of a tremendous amount of both public interest and media attention. As decisions that involve withholding or withdrawing life-prolonging treatment can impact on the length of a person's life a great deal of certainty must underpin these decisions. They must be made with the person's best interests at heart and have a robust LEP foundation.

To assist professionals in making these decisions, two important guidelines have been produced. The first guideline on withholding and withdrawing life-prolonging medical treatment (BMA, 2007) deals in detail with many of the issues that relate to decision making in this area. The second guideline has been jointly published by the BMA, the Resuscitation Council UK and the Royal Collage of Nursing (2007) and deals specifically with decisions that relate to cardiopulmonary resuscitation. Combined, these guidelines provide the most authoritative guidance on the subject for use with UK law and as such are essential reading for anyone involved in making, contributing to, or carrying out a decision to withhold life-prolonging medical treatment. In summary, these guidelines identify that that there are three separate circumstances where treatment can be withheld with legal and ethical justification. These are:

- When treatment will not be successful in achieving its aim
- When the burdens of treatment will be too much for the patient to endure
- When a patient with capacity for decision making does not want the treatment.

When considering for whom life-prolonging treatment would be of benefit and for whom it would be inappropriate, it is important to recognise that there are a number of decisions to be made. Some of these decisions are the responsibility of the healthcare team and others are the responsibility of the patient. When healthcare professionals are involved in making decisions, it is essential that these are based on an individual assessment of the patient's condition and circumstances. No patient should be prejudged as being inappropriate for treatment.

When treatment will not be successful in achieving its aim

The first point that needs to be identified is whether or not the proposed treatment will be effective in meeting its aim. If there is no realistic hope of success then the treatment should be withheld. In fact, it could easily be argued that if a treatment will not achieve it aims then in truth it is not a treatment at all. Where no evidence exists as to the usefulness of a treatment in a given clinical situation then justification for providing treatment is removed. While this assertion may cause concern over health professionals making decisions to 'give up' on patients when they are at their most vulnerable, in reality these decisions are no different from not offering an ineffective treatment in other circumstances. For example, making a decision to treat meningitis with aspirin would be seen as nonsensical as there is no evidence to support treating meningitis in this way, and if a health professional chose to treat a patient in such a way then they could well be questioned for providing a treatment that is destined to be unsuccessful. Examples of where resuscitative efforts are more than likely to fail are serious cerebrovascular accidents, metastatic cancer and septic shock.

When the burdens of treatment may be too much for the patient to endure

The second situation that needs to be considered involves a circumstance in which the proposed treatment may or may not be successful. Ethical consideration in this situation is needed when there is uncertainty of outcome, coupled with a proposed treatment that is likely to be intensive, possibly painful or uncomfortable and distressing to the patient. Another trigger for ethical consideration involves the question: Will the treatment, if successful in prolonging life, produce a life that is acceptable or unacceptable to the patient?

In this situation the decision is not solely a medical one. As medical success is a possibility, ethical justification for providing the treatment exists. The decision here becomes one that is concerned with patient autonomy and therefore any decision-making process must be shared with the patient and if appropriate their significant others. When uncertainty over outcome is a possibility, the patient should be central to the decision-making process. The patient who has the mental capacity for decision making should be given the opportunity to receive information about their condition, the proposed options available to them, what each of these options will involve and the medical implications of following each of the options. The information presented to the patient should be realistic in terms of likely outcomes. Judgement will need to be exercised as to how much information the patient needs to make a decision and the rate at which this can be imparted. Information should not be withheld by health professionals because they feel uncomfortable in having such discussions with patients. Research evidence shows that patients want to be involved in decisions about their lives.

When an adult patient with capacity for decision making does not want the treatment

The next point to consider is whether or not the patient wants the proposed treatment. Adult patients who have capacity for decision making have an absolute right to decide what will or will not happen to them, even if this decision is judged to be irrational or it will directly lead to their death in a reversible clinical situation. A good example of this would be a person who refuses blood or blood products on the grounds of religious beliefs, even if blood was judged to be essential to reverse major haemorrhage and save the person's life. If the person has the capacity to make the decision and they understand that refusing treatment may result in their death, nevertheless refusing treatment is an absolute right and one that should not be overruled.

Consent is a process through which a patient's wishes are established. For consent to be valid the person must:

- Have the mental capacity for decision making
- Be provided with information about the treatment options, their outcomes, risk and the outcome of non-treatment
- Be free from undue influence or duress in order to make their own decisions.

When the above criteria have been satisfied then it is a fundamental point of UK law that the patient's decision should be respected.

Occasionally, patients will request a treatment such as resuscitation where the medical team believes that it will be highly unlikely for success to follow the treatment. Health professionals are not obliged to provide a treatment requested by a patient if they feel it is clinically inappropriate. If this situation occurs it is useful to discuss the matter with the patient and establish what benefits the treatment will bring and why they feel it will be useful. Try to establish what the patient knows about the treatment and its success rates in the light of their current situation. It may be necessary to correct any misinformation that the patient has acquired and provide them with a realistic overview of their personal situation, explaining why the treatments would not work. If the patient is insistent on receiving a treatment that others feel is clinically inappropriate then it may be helpful to seek a second opinion, if the patient would find this useful.

Increasingly patients are making advanced decisions about how they would wish to be treated should they need a specific life-prolonging treatment. Many people are concerned that their wishes will not be upheld if they become unable to communicate or take part in decision making. This has caused an increasing number of people to write advanced directives. An advanced directive is a statement of the treatment that a person would accept or decline if a specific need arises. Advanced directives have legal standing if they are considered valid. For an advanced directive to be given validity it must satisfy the following criteria as identified by BMA et al. (2007).

- The patient was 18 years old or over and had capacity when the decision was made
- The decision is in writing, signed and witnessed
- It includes a statement that the advance decision is to apply even if the patient's life is at risk
- The advance decision has not been withdrawn
- The patient has not, since the advance decision was made, appointed a welfare attorney to make decisions about CPR on their behalf
- The patient has not done anything clearly inconsistent with its terms
- The circumstances that have arisen match those envisaged in the advance decision.

Where these criteria are satisfied then the patient's wishes must be followed.

People who lack mental capacity for decision making

If a patient lacks mental capacity for decision making then discussing treatment options and identifying how to proceed with either treatment or non-treatment can be complicated. The introduction of the Mental Capacity Act 2005 has brought about some significant changes to the way people who lose capacity for decision making can be treated. In the past, where a person lost capacity doctors would treat a patient in what they believed to be the patient's best interests. Post Mental Capacity Act 2005 the rules for surrogate decision making are stricter and new provisions have been introduced, such as the ability to appoint a person with lasting power of attorney who is able to make medical decisions on a patient's behalf should they lose capacity.

The first point that needs to be made is that when considering mental capacity it is presumed that each and every adult has capacity unless it can be proven otherwise. When a person's capacity for decision making is called into doubt, there are two questions that need to be asked as part of an assessment: 'Is there an impairment of, or disturbance of the person's mind or brain?', and, if the answer to this question is 'Yes', then the second question serves to establish 'If the impairment or disturbance is sufficient to cause the person to be unable to make a decision at the relevant time' (Department of Health, 2007). If the person is judged to lack capacity for decision making then an alternative way of making decisions about care will be needed. Details of the options for decision making in these circumstance are included in the Department of Health's 2007 publication *Mental Capacity Act 2005 Core Training Set*.

Documenting treatment decisions

Once a decision has been made it is necessary to communicate this to the whole team that is caring for the person. This will involve a comprehensive record in the notes that provides a justification for the decision and details of how involved the patient has been. If the decision relates to the withholding of CPR then a 'Do Not Attempt Resuscitation' (DNAR) form is completed in most hospitals. Many hospitals use a standard form to record these decisions. Once completed, this form is placed in a prominent location within the notes. In order that the decision is upheld when patient care is transferred, say to another department or to an ambulance, then the receiving health professionals should be made aware of the document and the decision.

Limits of DNAR decisions and circumstances where DNAR decisions may not apply

The presence of a DNAR decision is specific to CPR. A patient who is the subject of a DNAR decision should receive all other treatment that is indicated and that they have consented to. DNAR decisions are context-specific; for example, if a person with a malignancy makes a DNAR decision it is likely that the decision is made to cover cardiac arrest which is precipitated by an end-stage malignant condition. If the person, while relatively well, was to choke and suffer a respiratory arrest then this is outside of the context that the initial decision was made in. As airway obstruction is an eminently reversible condition justification would exist for instigating resuscitation in this circumstance as it is distinct from the circumstances that were anticipated.

Conclusion

Acutely ill patients present with a range of LEP issues that health professionals will have to address at some time in their practice. Holding a knowledge of the basic LEP issues that underpin the practice of acute care will assist tremendously when used by a critically thinking professional. While many of the LEP issues that relate to the care of the acutely ill are common to all areas of healthcare, the decision to withhold or withdraw life-sustaining medical treatment is of particular importance to practitioners in this area.

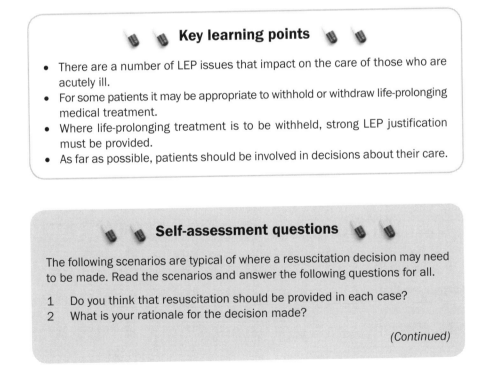

Key learning points

- There are a number of LEP issues that impact on the care of those who are acutely ill.
- For some patients it may be appropriate to withhold or withdraw life-prolonging medical treatment.
- Where life-prolonging treatment is to be withheld, strong LEP justification must be provided.
- As far as possible, patients should be involved in decisions about their care.

Self-assessment questions

The following scenarios are typical of where a resuscitation decision may need to be made. Read the scenarios and answer the following questions for all.

1 Do you think that resuscitation should be provided in each case?
2 What is your rationale for the decision made?

(Continued)

(Continued)

Case 1

A 53-year-old man with type 1 diabetes is admitted to hospital after suffering a ventricular fibrillation arrest in the presence of paramedics. He was defibrillated twice and received two minutes of CPR. By the time he had arrived at hospital he was responsive to voice.

Case 2

A 62-year-old woman with ovarian cancer develops a temperature of 39.0°C despite being on appropriate antibiotics. Her blood pressure is 76/34 mmHg. Fluid challenges have failed to raise her blood pressure as have vasopressors. Sepsis has been presumed as the diagnosis.

Case 3

A 98-year-old woman, who lives independently at home with her husband, was admitted to hospital for intravenous antibiotics to treat cellulitis. After receiving her second dose she has anaphylaxis and has a ventricular fibrillation arrest.

Discussion

Case 1

This man has had primary cardiac arrest and responded well to prompt treatment. There is no reason to believe that he would not respond equally well to further treatment should he have another arrest. Resuscitation should be provided in this case unless the man has registered his objection to being treated in this way.

Case 2

This woman is in a grave condition. Patients with sepsis and cancer often do not do well following resuscitation. Maximal medical therapy has been attempted in this patient's case and it has failed to reverse the shock. It is likely to be appropriate to withhold resuscitation in this case.

Case 3

While this woman is relatively old, the cause of her arrest is potentially reversible. Her quality of life seems to be good prior to her arrest and as such justification for providing treatment is present. Denying this person treatment solely on the basis of age will be unethical and likely to be unlawful.

Further reading

British Medical Association (2007) *Withholding and Withdrawing Life-Prolonging Medical Treatment*, 3rd edn. London: BMA & Blackwell Publishing.

This detailed guide looks at the LEP issues that surround the withholding and withdrawing of all treatments that are potentially life-prolonging. Its logical approach makes this a practically useful guide.

British Medical Association, Resuscitation Council UK and Royal Collage of Nursing (2007) *Decisions Relating to Cardiopulmonary Resuscitation*. London: British Medical Association, Resuscitation Council UK, Royal Collage of Nursing.
This is an important guideline that addresses how decisions relating to CPR should be made, documented and reviewed.

Department of Health (2007) *Mental Capacity Act 2005 Core Training Set*. London: Department of Health.
This document provides a readable introduction to the provisions of the Mental Capacity Act 2005.

References

Adam, S. and Osborne, S. (2005) *Critical Care Nursing Science and Practice*. Oxford: Oxford University Press.

Audit Commission (1999) *Critical to Success. The Place of Efficient and Effective Critical Care Services within the Acute Hospital*. London: Audit Commission Publications.

BBC (2005) *Mobile 999 Contact Idea Spreads*. London: BBC. Online 2, http://news.bbc.co.uk/1/hi/england/4674331stm (accessed 1 Aug 2010).

Beckett, G., Walker, S., Rae, P. and Ashby, P. (2005) *Lecture Notes: Clinical Biochemistry*, 7th edn. Oxford: Blackwell Publishing.

Berry, A. and Stevens, A. (2008) 'Aiming to save lives', *Critical Care*, 12 (Suppl. 2): 426.

Bourke, S.J. (2007) *Lecture Notes on Respiratory Medicine*. Oxford: Blackwell Publishing.

British Hypertension Society (2004) *Validated Blood Pressure Monitors*. London: British Hypertension Society. Online, http://www.bhsoc.org/blood_pressure_list.stm (accessed 10 October 2010).

British Medical Association (2007) *Withholding and Withdrawing Life-Prolonging Medical Treatment*, 3rd edn. London: BMA & Blackwell Publishing.

British Medical Association, Resuscitation Council UK and Royal Collage of Nursing (2007) *Decisions Relating to Cardiopulmonary Resuscitation*. London: British Medical Association, Resuscitation Council UK and Royal Collage of Nursing.

British Thoracic Society and Scottish Intercollegiate Guideline Network (2008) *British Guideline on the Management of Asthma: A National Clinical Guideline*. London: BTS. Online: www.brit-thoracic.org.uk.

Brooker, C. (1998) *Human Structure and Function*, 2nd edn. London: Mosby.

Caldicott, F. (1997) *Report on the Review of Patient-Identifiable Information*. London: Department of Health.

Clancy, J. and McVicar, A. (2009) *Physiology and Anatomy for Nurses and Healthcare Practitioners: A Homeostatic Approach*. London: Hodder Arnold.

Cohen, J. (2009) 'Interrater reliability and predictive validity of the FOUR score coma scale in a pediatric population', *Journal of Neuroscience Nursing*, 41 (5): 261–7.

Cooper, N., Forrest, K. and Cramp, P. (2006) *Essential Guide to Acute Care*, 2nd edn. Oxford: Blackwell Publishing & BMJ Books.

Dellinger, R.P., Levy, M.M. and Carlet, J.M. et al. (2008) 'Surviving Sepsis Campaign: International guidelines for management of severe sepsis and septic shock: 2008 [published correction appears in *Crit Care Med* 2008; 36:1394–1396]', *Critical Care Medicine* 36: 296–327.

Department of Health (2007) *Mental Capacity Act 2005 Core Training Set*. London: Department of Health.

Department of Health (2008) *Critical Care Census, NHS Organisations in England, January 2008*. London: Department of Health.

Diamond, J. (2004) *C: Because Cowards Get Cancer Too*. London: Random House.

Eaton, J. (1999) *Essentials of Immediate Medical Care*. London: Churchill Livingstone.

Eberle, B., Dick, W.F., Schneider, T., Wisser, G., Doetsch, S. and Tzanova, I. (1996) 'Checking the carotid pulse check: diagnostic accuracy of first responders in patients with and without a pulse', *Resuscitation*, 33 (2): 107–16.

Epstein, O., Perkin, D., Cookson, J. and de Bono, D. (2003) *Clinical Examination*, 3rd edn. Edinburgh: Mosby.

Faulkner, A. (2000) 'Communication with patients families, and other professionals', in M. Fallon and B. O'Neil (eds), *ABC of Palliative Care*. London: BMJ Books.

Franklin, C. and Mathew, J. (1994) 'Developing strategies to prevent in-hospital cardiac arrest: analyzing responses of physicians and nurses in the hours before the event', *Critical Care Medicine*, 22: 244–7.

Gill, M., Reiley, D. and Green, S. (2004) 'Interrater reliability of Glasgow Coma Scale scores in the emergency department', *Annals of Emergency Medicine*, 43 (2): 215–23.

Gray, H., Dawkins, K., Morgan, J. and Simpson, I. (2008) *Lecture Notes: Cardiology*. Oxford: Blackwell Publishing.

Greenbank, A. (2003) *The Book of Survival: The Original Guide to Staying Alive in the City, the Suburbs and the Wild Lands Beyond*. New York: Hatherleigh Press.

Hamilton, R. (2005) 'Nurses' knowledge and skill retention following cardiopulmonary resuscitation training: a review of the literature', *Journal of Advanced Nursing*, 51 (3): 288–97.

Hampton, J.R. (2003) *The ECG Made Easy*. London: Churchill Livingstone.

Handley, A., Koster, R., Monsieurs, K., Perkins, D., Davies, S. and Bossaert, L. (2005) 'European Resuscitation Council Guidelines for Resuscitation 2005; Section 2. Adult basic life support and use of automated external defibrillators', *Resuscitation*, 67S1: S7–23.

Harrison, D.A., Brady, A.R. and Rowan, K. (2004) 'Case mix, outcome and length of stay for admissions to adult, general critical care units in England, Wales and Northern Ireland: the Intensive Care National Audit & Research Centre Case Mix Programme Database', *Critical Care*, 8: R99–R111.

Harrison, R. and Daly, L. (2006) *Acute Medical Emergencies: A Nursing Guide*. Edinburgh: Churchill Livingstone.

Health Professions Council (2008) *Standards of Conduct, Performance and Ethics*. London: Health Professions Council.

HM Government (2008) *Information Sharing Guidance for Practitioners and Managers*. London: Department for Children, Schools and Families and Department for Communities and Local Government.

Hodgetts, T.J., Kenward, G., Vlackonikolis, I., Payne, S., Castle, N., Crouch, R., Ineson, N. and Shaikh, L. (2002) 'Incidence, location and reasons for avoidable in-hospital cardiac arrest in a district general hospital', *Resuscitation*, 54:115–23.

Holdgate, A., Asha, S., Craig, J. and Thompson, J. (2003) 'Comparison of a verbal numeric rating scale with the visual analogue scale for the measurement of acute pain', *Emergency Medicine*, 15 (5–6): 441–6.

International Liaison Committee on Resuscitation (2010) Worksheets 2010. International Liaison Committee on Resuscitation. Online, http://www.ilcor.org/en/consensus-2010/worksheets-2010/ (accessed 31 July 2010).

Jenkins, R.D. and Gerred, S.J. (2005) *ECGs by Example*. London: Churchill Livingstone.

Juarcz, V.J. and Lyons, M. (1996) 'Interrater reliability of the Glasgow Coma Scale', *Journal of Neuroscience Nursing*, 28 (4): 213–14.

Kaye, W., Rallis, S.F., Mancini, M.E., Linhares, K.C., Angell, M.L., Donovan, D.S., Zajano, N.C. and Finger, J.A. (1991) 'The problem of poor retention of cardiopulmonary resuscitation skills may lie with the instructor, not the learner or the curriculum', *Resuscitation*, 21 (1): 67–87.

Kübler-Ross, E. (1973) *On Death and Dying*. Sussex: Routledge.

Laerdal Medical (2010) *The Circle of Learning*. Kent: Laerdal Medical. Online: http://www.laerdal.info/doc/6732687/The-Circle-of-Learning.html (accessed 11 August 2010).

Lakhanin, S., Dilly, D., Finlayson, C. and Dogan, A. (2003) *Basic Pathology: An Introduction to the Mechanisms of Disease*. London: Hodder Arnold.

Leah, V. and Coats, T.J. (1999) 'In-hospital resuscitation – what should we be teaching?', *Resuscitation*, 41 (2): 197–83.

McLauchlan, C. (2000) 'Handling distressed relatives and breaking bad news', in P. Driscoll, D. Skinner and R. Earlam (eds), *ABC of Major Trauma*. London: Wiley-Blackwell.

McQuillan, P., Pilkington, S., Allan, A., Taylor, B., Short, A., Morgan, G., Nielsen, M., Barrett, D., Smith, G. and Collins, C.H. (1998) 'Confidential inquiry into quality of care before admission to intensive care', *BMJ*, 316: 1853–8.

Morgan, R.J.M., Williams, F. and Wright, M.M. (1997) 'An early warning scoring system for detecting developing critical illness', *Clinical Intensive Care*, 8: 100.

Moss, B. (2008) *Communication Skills for Health & Social Care*. London: Sage Publications.

Moule, P. (2000) 'Checking the carotid pulse: diagnostic accuracy in students of the healthcare professions', *Resuscitation*, 44 (3): 195–201.

National Collaborating Centre for Chronic Conditions (2006) *Atrial Fibrillation: National Clinical Guideline for Management in Primary and Secondary Care*. London: Royal College of Physicians.

National Confidential Enquiry into Patient Outcome and Death (2005) *An Acute Problem. A Report of the National Confidential Enquiry into Patient Outcome and Death*. London: NCEPOD.

National Institute for Health and Clinical Excellence (2007) *Acutely Ill Patients in Hospital; Recognition of and Response to Acute Illness in Adults in Hospital*. London: NICE.

Nolan, J. and Baskett, P. (eds) (2005) 'European Resuscitation Council Guidelines for Resuscitation 2005', *Resuscitation*, 67 (Suppl.): S1–S189.

Nolan, J.P., Deakin, C.D., Soar, J., Bottiger, B.W. and Smith G. (2005) 'European Resuscitation Council Guidelines for Resuscitation 2005, Section 4, Adult Advanced Life Support', *Resuscitation*, 67 (Suppl.): S39–S86.

Nursing and Midwifery Council (2008) *The Code, Standards of Conduct, Performance and Ethics for Nurses and Midwives*. London: Nursing and Midwifery Council.

O'Brien, E., Asmar, R., Beilin, L., Imai, Y., Mallion, J., Mancia, G., Mengden, T., Myers, M., Padfield, P., Palatini, P., Parati, G., Pickering, T., Redon, J., Staessen, J., Stergiou, G. and Verdecchia, P. on behalf of the European Society of Hypertension Working Group on Blood Pressure Monitoring. (2003) 'European Society of Hypertension recommendations for conventional, ambulatory and home blood pressure measurement', *Journal of Hypertension*, 21: 821–48.

O'Donnell, C. (1990) 'A survey of opinion amongst trained nurses and junior medical staff on current practices in resuscitation', *Journal of Advanced Nursing*, 15: 1175–80.

O'Driscoll, B., Howard, L. and Davison, A. on behalf of the British Thoracic Society Emergency Oxygen Guideline Development Group, a subgroup of the British Thoracic Society Standards of Care Committee. (2008) 'Guideline for emergency oxygen use in adult patients', *Thorax*, 63 (Suppl. VI).

Office for National Statistics (2004) *Mortality Statistics Cause, Review of the Registrar General on Deaths by Cause, Sex and Age, in England and Wales*, London: HMSO.

Peberdy, M.A., Kaye, W., Ornato, J.P., Larkin, G.L., Nadkarni, V., Mancini, M.E., Berg, R.A., Nichol, G. and Lane-Trultt, T. (2003) 'Cardiopulmonary resuscitation of adults in the hospital: A report of 14720 cardiac arrests from the National Registry of Cardiopulmonary Resuscitation', *Resuscitation*, 58 (3): 297–308.

Popcock, G. and Richards, C.D. (2006) *Human Physiology: The Basis of Medicine*, 3rd edn. Oxford: Oxford University Press.

Prytherch, D., Smith, G., Schmidt, P. and Featherstone, P. (2010) 'ViEWS – towards a national early warning score for detecting adult in-patient deterioration', *Resuscitation*, 81: 932–7.

Rang, H.P., Dale, M.M., Ritter, J.M. and Flower, R.J. (2007) *Rang and Dale's Pharmacology*, 6th edn. Edinburgh: Churchill Livingstone.

Resuscitation Council UK (2010) *Resuscitation Guidelines 2010*. London: Resuscitation Council UK.

Resuscitation Council (UK) and Intercollegiate Board for Training in Intensive Care Medicine (2005) *Acute Care in Undergraduate Teaching (ACUTE) Initiative*. London: Resuscitation Council UK.

Resuscitation Council UK (2008) *Emergency Treatment of Anaphylactic Reactions: Guidelines for Healthcare Providers*. London: Resuscitation Council UK.

Rivers, E., Nguyen, B., Havstad, S., Ressler, J., Muzzin, A., Knoblich, B., Peterson, E. and Tomlanovich, M. for the Early Goal-Directed Therapy Collaborative Group (2001) 'Early goal-directed therapy in the treatment of severe sepsis and septic shock', *New England Journal of Medicine*, 345 (19): 1368–77.

Royal College of Physicians (2007) *Acute Medical Care: The Right Person, in the Right Setting – First Time*. London: Royal College of Physicians.

Royal College of Physicians (2008) *Non-Invasive Ventilation in Chronic Obstructive Pulmonary Disease: Management of Type 2 Respiratory Failure*. London: Royal College of Physicians.

Rutishauser, S. (1999) *Physiology and Anatomy: A Basis for Nursing and Healthcare*. Edinburgh: Churchill Livingstone.

Sheldon, F. (2000) 'Bereavement', in M. Fallon and B. O'Neil (eds), *ABC of Palliative Care*. London: BMJ Books.

Smith, G.B., Osgood, V.M. and Crane, S., ALERT™ Course Development Group (2002) 'ALERT™ – A Multiprofessional training course in the care of the acutely ill adult patient', *Resuscitation*, 52 (3): 281–6.

Soar, J., Perkins, G.D., Harris, S. and Nolan, J. for Immediate Life Support Working Group Resuscitation Council (UK) (2003) 'The immediate life support course', *Resuscitation*, 57 (1): 21–6.

Steane, A. (2007) *Who Cares? One Family's Shocking Story of Care in Today's NHS*. Bournemouth: Original Book Co.

Stubbe, C.P., Kruger, M., Rutherford, P. and Gemmell, L. (2001) 'Validation of a modified early warning score in medical admissions', *Quarterly Journal of Medicine*, 94: 521–6.

Sulmasy, D.P., Terry, P.B., Weismann, C.S., Miller, D.J., Stallings, R.Y., Vettese, M.A. and Haller, K.B. (1998) 'The accuracy of substituted judgements in patients with terminal diagnoses', *Annals of Internal Medicine*, 128 (8): 621–9.

Teasdale, G. and Jennett, B. (1974) 'Assessment of coma and impaired consciousness. A practical scale', *Lancet*, ii: 81–4.

Tibballs, J. and Russell, P. (2009) 'Reliability of pulse palpation by healthcare personnel to diagnose paediatric cardiac arrest', *Resuscitation*, 80 (1): 61–4.

Tortora, G.J. and Nielsen, M.T. (2009) *Principles of Human Anatomy*, 11th edn. Oxford: John Wiley & Sons.

Index

NOTE: Page numbers in *italic type* refer to figures and tables.

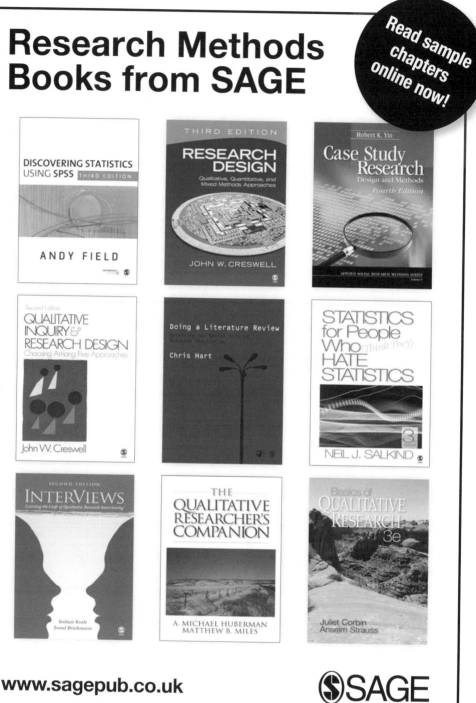

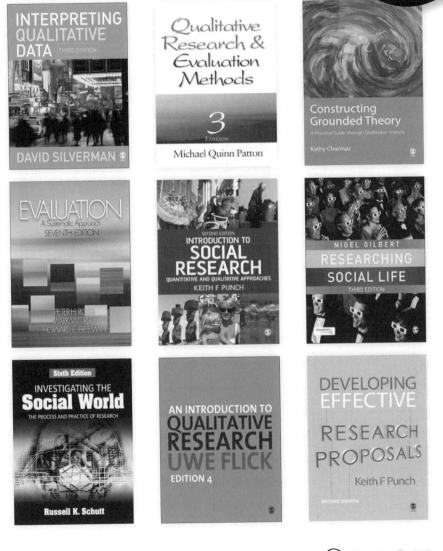
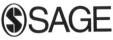

Exciting Education Texts from SAGE

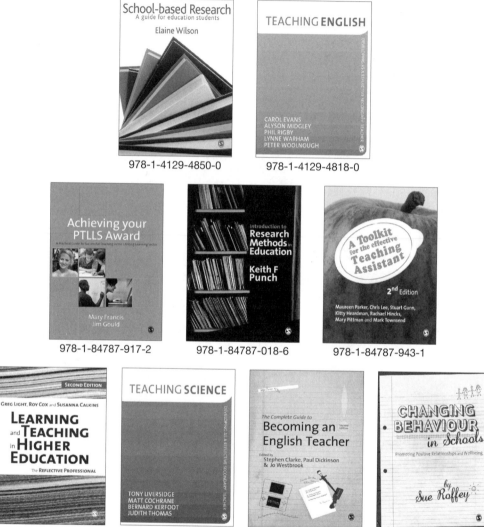

School-based Research
A guide for education students
Elaine Wilson
978-1-4129-4850-0

TEACHING ENGLISH
CAROL EVANS
ALYSON MIDGLEY
PHIL RIGBY
LYNNE WARHAM
PETER WOOLNOUGH
978-1-4129-4818-0

Achieving your PTLLS Award
A Practical Guide to Successful Teaching in the Lifelong Learning Sector
Mary Francis
Jim Gould
978-1-84787-917-2

Introduction to Research Methods in Education
Keith F Punch
978-1-84787-018-6

A Toolkit for the effective Teaching Assistant
2nd Edition
Maureen Parker, Chris Lee, Stuart Gunn,
Kitty Heardman, Rachael Hincks,
Mary Pittman and Mark Townsend
978-1-84787-943-1

SECOND EDITION
GREG LIGHT, ROY COX and SUSANNA CALKINS
LEARNING and TEACHING in HIGHER EDUCATION
The REFLECTIVE PROFESSIONAL
978-1-84860-008-9

TEACHING SCIENCE
TONY LIVERSIDGE
MATT COCHRANE
BERNARD KERFOOT
JUDITH THOMAS
978-1-84787-362-0

The Complete Guide to Becoming an English Teacher Second Edition
Edited by
Stephen Clarke, Paul Dickinson
& Jo Westbrook
978-1-84787-289-0

CHANGING BEHAVIOUR in Schools
Promoting Positive Relationships and Wellbeing
by Sue Roffey
978-1-84920-078-3

Find out more about these titles and our wide range of books for education students and practitioners at **www.sagepub.co.uk/education**

$\bigodot$SAGE